Handbook of
Small Animal Dentistry
Second Edition

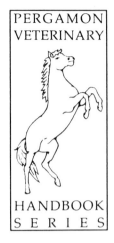

Handbook of
Small Animal Dentistry
Second Edition

Peter Emily

Director of Animal Dentistry, Colorado State University

and

Susanna Penman

Founding President, British Veterinary Dental Association

PERGAMON PRESS

OXFORD · NEW YORK · SEOUL · TOKYO

U.K.	Pergamon Press Ltd, Headington Hill Hall, Oxford OX3 0BW, England
U.S.A.	Pergamon Press Inc, 660 White Plains Road, Tarrytown, New York 10591-5153, U.S.A.
KOREA	Pergamon Press Korea, KPO Box 315, Seoul 110-603, Korea
JAPAN	Pergamon Press Japan, Tsunashima Building Annex, 3-20-12 Yushima, Bunkyo-ku, Tokyo 113, Japan

First edition 1990
Second edition 1994

Library of Congress Cataloging in Publication Data
Handbook of small animal dentistry/by Peter Emily and Susanna Penman. 2nd ed.
p. cm. (Pergamon veterinary handbook series)
Includes index.
1. Veterinary dentistry Handbooks, manuals, etc. 2. Dogs-Diseases Handbooks, manuals, etc. 3. Cats-Diseases Handbooks, manuals, etc. I. Penman, Susanna. II. Title III. Series.
SF992.M68E45 1994
636.089'76 dc20

British Library Cataloguing in Publication Data
A catalogue record for this book is available from the British Library

ISBN 0 08 042287 X Flexicover
ISBN 0 08 042291 8 Hardcover

The line drawings in this book have been designed by Maurizia Merati.
The following figures were drawn by Maurizia Merati and are reproduced with her permission: Figs 1.1, 1.2, 1.3, 1.4, 1.5, 2.3, 4.4, 4.5, 4.6, 4.7, 4.8, 4.9.

Printed in Great Britain by BPCC Wheatons Limited, Exeter

Contents

Preface to the First Edition

The object of its handbook is to give practical guidance to the treatment of the dental conditions encountered daily in veterinary practice. It is written for the veterinary practitioner and student as a working manual, with emphasis on the practical aspects. The procedures most frequently used in small animal dentistry are described in a detailed step-by-step approach, with numerous drawings and photographs to illustrate the important points and the instrumentation required. The layout of the pages describing the techniques has been carefully designed to be clear and easy to use, with detailed descriptions and illustrations. The book is specially bound so that when open it can lie flat on a table to facilitate its use.

The clarity and accuracy of the illustrations are of paramount importance in a book of this kind. We are most grateful to Maurizia Merati and Adam Harras for their time, effort and attention to detail in the production of the drawings. Mr and Mrs Sweeney very kindly lent us six chinchilla skulls exhibiting the various stages of anaesognathism and root protrusion, which enabled us to illustrate this particular malocclusion more clearly. Our thanks are also due to Shor-line, Henry Schein Inc., and Baxter Veterinary for providing photographs of equipment. Marion Jowett and Andrew Edney have been wonderful editors; we have all enjoyed working together as a team.

As veterinary dentistry is evolving at such a rate, a second edition will no doubt soon be required. Please send your comments and queries to Dr P. Emily, 1051 Independence Street, Lakewood, CO 80215, USA, or Ms S. Penman, 29 Upper Bourne Lane, Farnham, Surrey GU10 4RG, UK.

Susanna Penman, BVSC, MRCVS
Peter Emily, DDS

Preface to the Second Edition

Since the first edition of the *Handbook of Small Animal Dentistry* was published, veterinary dentistry has developed into a major speciality. It is now taught in more detail in numerous veterinary schools, where this book is used extensively, and many veterinary practitioners have begun to specialize in dentistry. This second edition has been produced as a response to recent developments in materials and techniques, and to readers' comments. We have also taken the opportunity to correct the few small errors which somehow crept into the first edition.

During the last four years, our knowledge of certain conditions has increased. There is now a different, more thorough approach to the treatment of feline subgingival resorptive lesions. Immature teeth with necrotic pulps can be induced to continue their development if they are treated correctly. It is possible to extract the incisors of small domestic herbivores without great difficulty. The techniques for these and more conditions are described in the detailed step-by-step approach which has proved so easy to follow.

New equipment has evolved to satisfy the demands of the veterinary dental specialist. Ultrasonic scalers with irrigation through the tip can be used subgingivally. An oscillating polishing cup is now available which eliminates the problem of hair winding onto the polishing head. The use of the rotosonic scaler is more strongly discouraged.

Dental materials are constantly changing, with new products arriving at a prodigious rate. Several adhesives have been developed to bond amalgam to tooth structure. Light-cured glass-ionomers are now available, which make glass-ionomers much easier to use.

We are most grateful to the readers who sent in comments and particularly to Cecilia Gorrel, David Crossley and John Robinson for their help in the production of this second edition. We would also like to thank Steve Haynes for all of his work on the illustrations in this edition.

Susanna Penman, BVSC, MRCVS
Peter Emily, DDS

1
Anatomy

Head Shapes

The shape of the head affects the positioning of teeth and hence their relationship and predisposition to disease.

Dog

There is considerable variation between breeds, with three major types:

Dolichocephalic: long, narrow muzzle, e.g. Borzoi, Dobermann, Greyhound, Saluki
Mesaticephalic: medium length and width of muzzle, e.g. Labrador Retriever, German Shepherd Dog, most spaniels, terriers and hounds; 75% of dogs are mesaticephalic
Brachycephalic: short wide muzzle, commonly with reverse scissor bite e.g. Pekingese, Pug, Boxer, Shih Tzu, Bulldog.

Cat

The shape of cats' heads is more uniform, but some breeds are selected for their brachycephalic characteristics, e.g. Persians, or their long skulls, e.g. Orientals.

Occlusal Relationships

Normal Occlusion

The normal bite of an adult dog is shown in Fig. 1.1. It is characterized by:

- the scissor bite of the incisors; the upper incisors are just rostral to the lower incisors; the incisal tips of the lower incisors contact the cingula and cusps of the upper incisors

- the interdigitation of the canines: the lower canine crown lies exactly between the upper lateral incisor and the upper canine, touching neither
- the 'pinking shear' effect of the premolars: the tips of their crowns oppose the interdental spaces of the opposite arcade, the lower first premolar being the most rostral.

The articulation of the jaws of the carnivore is designed to produce the maximum biting force, restricting the jaw movement to the vertical plane. Hence the teeth (mostly the premolars) can be precisely arranged for shearing and cutting. The biting force exerted in the dog is approximately 1200 pounds per square inch, compared with 150 pounds per square inch in man.

Malocclusions

Any deviation from the above constitutes some degree of malocclusion (Fig. 1.2). Some breed standards allow certain malocclusions as part of the characteristics of the breed, notably the reverse scissor or prognathic bite of the brachycephalic breeds.

Briefly, the malocclusions are as follows.

Mandibular brachygnathism (overshot)

The maxilla is too long relative to the mandible. The degree of brachygnathism varies, the malocclusion showing the following characteristics:

- the upper incisors are more rostral to the lower incisors than normal (by 0.5 mm to 5 cm or more), preventing the lower incisors from touching the cingula of their upper counterparts

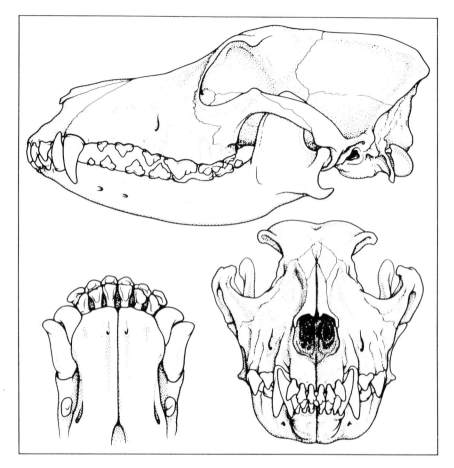

Fɪɢ. 1.1 The normal bite of an adult dog. Top: Lateral view of the skull showing the interdigitation of the canines and the pinking shear effect of the premolars. Bottom left: Ventral view of the rostral section of the skull, showing the scissor bite of the incisors. Bottom right: Rostral view of the skull showing that the mandible is narrower than the maxilla.

- the upper canines are in various rostral deviations: caudal to but touching the lower canines (mild brachygnathism); level with the lower canines; rostral to the lower canines (more severe brachygnathism)
- the upper premolars are rostrally displaced relative to the lower premolars, disrupting the 'pinking shear' effect: the degree of displacement is similar to that of the incisors and canines.

Mandibular prognathism (undershot)

The mandible is too long relative to the maxilla. The degree of prognathism varies as follows:

- the lower canines touch the upper lateral incisors; the incisor occlusion is often normal; the mandibular premolars are usually rostrally displaced, disrupting the 'pinking shear' effect
- level bite: the upper and lower incisors meet at their incisal edges, resulting in excessive attrition; the lower canines are often touching the upper lateral incisors; the mandibular premolars are usually rostrally displaced
- reverse scissor bite: the lower incisors are rostral to the upper incisors by 0.5 mm to 5 cm or more; the lower canines may be caudal to but touching the upper lateral incisors, or may be rostral to the upper lateral incisors; the mandibular premolars are rostrally displaced to a similar degree.

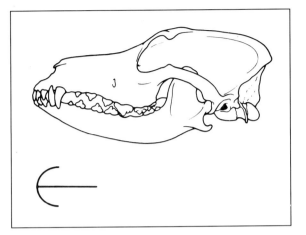

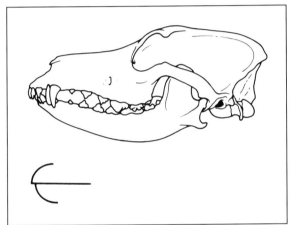

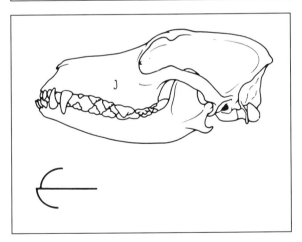

FIG. 1.2 Occlusion and malocclusions: lateral view of skulls with diagrams representing the lip shapes. Top: Normal, class I bite. Centre: Brachygnathic, class II bite, also known as retrusive or overshot. Bottom: Prognathic, class III bite, also known as protrusive or undershot.

Wry bite

One side of the mandible or maxilla or one side of the head grows more than the other side, producing a malocclusion of varying degree. In its mildest form, a one-sided prognathic or brachygnathic bite may develop, with an apparently normal skull. In more severe cases, a crooked head and bite, both with a deviated midline and an open bite may develop (Fig. 1.3).

Open bite

An anterior open bite is seen in the incisors, often in conjunction with a wry bite. Affected teeth are displaced vertically and do not occlude normally (Fig. 1.3). The space between the upper and lower incisors can vary from 0.5 mm to 2.0 cm.

A posterior open bite affects the premolars. It may occur when a strong dental interlock prevents the formation of a genetically induced mandibular prognathism, so that the extra mandibular length is accommodated by ventral or lateral bowing of the mandible. A wry bite may also include a posterior open bite.

Anterior crossbite

In this condition, some of the upper incisors are caudal to their lower counterparts (if the three adjacent incisors of one side are involved, it may be a wry bite). In some cases, this is thought to be the result of retained deciduous incisors; however, affected animals often seem to develop a prognathic bite, so an anterior crossbite seen in an immature animal may be the first signs of a developing prognathism.

Base narrow mandibular canines

The mandible is too narrow relative to the maxilla. Unless the lower canines flare out considerably, they will impinge on the hard palate. Retained deciduous lower canines can cause this malocclusion with a mandible of normal width, and can exacerbate it with a narrow mandible.

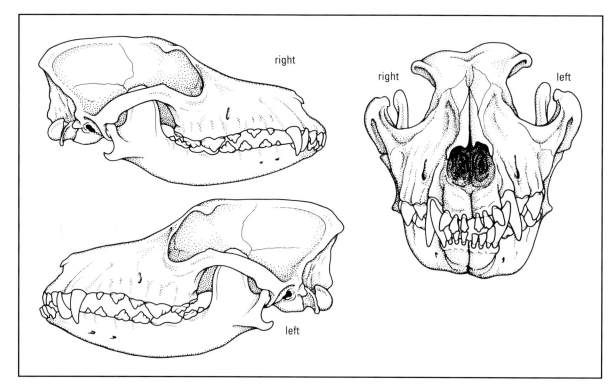

FIG. 1.3 Wry bite. Top left: Right lateral view of the skull showing a normal occlusion. Bottom left: Left lateral view of the skull showing a prognathic and open bite. Right: Rostral view of the skull showing deviation of the midline (upper incisors towards the overdeveloped side), the premolar open bite and the overdevelopment of the left side of the skull.

Correction

Correcting hereditary malocclusions is unacceptable unless the animal is neutered, in common with any correctable inherited condition. The inheritance of conditions secondary to retained deciduous teeth is debatable, as is their correction. Malocclusions causing trauma and pain should be corrected by orthodontics, tooth shortening and pulpotomy, or extraction. Prevention is preferable; retained deciduous teeth should be extracted as soon as possible.

Dentition

Teeth are categorized according to their function:

Incisors: cutting, nibbling, delicate work
6 in each jaw
small, single-rooted teeth.

Canines: holding, tearing
2 in each jaw
the largest, strongest, single-rooted teeth.

Premolars: cutting, holding, shearing
dog: 8 in each jaw
cat: 6 in the maxilla, 4 in the mandible
single-, double- and triple-rooted.

Molars: grinding
dog: 4 in the maxilla, 6 in the mandible
cat: 2 in each jaw
single-, double- and triple-rooted.

Although dogs and cats are both classed zoologically as carnivores, dogs are more omnivorous than cats and hence require more grinding molars. The lower first molars in dogs and cats are also involved in premolar activities; their classification is therefore debatable. 'Carnassial' teeth are the largest cutting teeth. These are the upper fourth premolars and

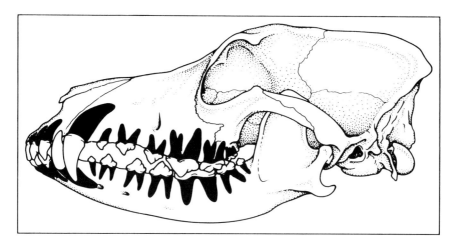

FIG. 1.4 Lateral view of the skull of an adult dog, showing the sizes and positions of the teeth and their roots, in normal occlusion.

lower first molars in dogs and the upper third premolars and lower molars in cats. Figures 1.4 and 1.5 show the normal occlusion of the dog and cat, with the shapes, sizes and position of the teeth and their roots relative to the skull, jawbones and crowns.

Dental Formula

The classification of teeth can be recorded as a dental formula which shows the number of teeth in the upper and lower jaws of one side of the head.

Dog: Temporary teeth $2(I\frac{3}{3} C\frac{1}{1} P\frac{3}{3})$ = 28

 Permanent teeth $2(I\frac{3}{3} C\frac{1}{1} P\frac{4}{4} M\frac{2}{3})$ = 42

Cat: Temporary teeth $2(I\frac{3}{3} C\frac{1}{1} P\frac{3}{2})$ = 26

 Permanent teeth $2(I\frac{3}{3} C\frac{1}{1} P\frac{3}{2} M\frac{1}{1})$ = 30

'I' represents incisors, 'C' represents canines, 'P' represents premolars, 'M' represents molars; ' $\frac{3}{2}$ ' represents 2 upper molars and 3 lower molars on one side.

Not all permanent teeth are preceded by temporary teeth, because when the temporaries erupt, the head is not big enough to accommodate the full number.

Eruption of Temporary and Permanent Teeth

Eruption Times

Puppies and kittens are not born with teeth. Their temporary (deciduous, milk or baby)

teeth start to erupt when they are about 3 weeks old. The permanent teeth replace their temporary counterparts gradually, from about 3 months of age, as shown in Fig.1.6.

The crowns of the permanent teeth are formed by approximately 11 weeks of age, but

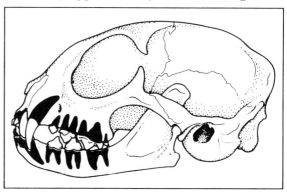

FIG. 1.5 Lateral view of the skull of an adult cat, showing the sizes and positions of the teeth and their roots, in normal occlusion.

THE APPROXIMATE AGES OF DOGS AND CATS (IN WEEKS) WHEN TEETH ERUPT			
	Temporary teeth		Permanent teeth
	Puppy	Kitten	Dog	Cat
Incisors	4–6	3–4	12–16	11–16
Canines	3–5	3–4	12–20	12–20
Premolars	5–6	5–6	16–20	16–20
Molars	–	–	20–24	20–24

FIG. 1.6 The approximate ages of dogs and cats (in weeks) when teeth erupt.

remain hidden within the jawbone. As their roots develop, so the crowns erupt through the gingiva. The proximity of the erupting crown to the root of the temporary tooth contributes to the resorption of the root. The temporary tooth is then lost, providing a clear pathway for the erupting permanent tooth. Ideally, the temporary tooth should be lost as the permanent crown erupts through the gingiva.

Retained Temporary Teeth

Any temporary tooth remaining in place after the erupting permanent tooth has emerged through the gingiva should be removed under general anaesthesia. Left in place, retained temporary teeth usually cause malocclusions and localized gingivitis. Debris trapped between the two teeth produces the gingivitis. The malocclusions are the result of the deviation of the erupting tooth's pathway enforced by the presence of the temporary tooth. The smaller breeds are most often affected by this condition which seems to be familial, although the exact degree and mode of inheritance are not known. The three most frequently affected areas are the lower canines, the upper canines and the incisors.

Lower canines

The lower permanent canine begins eruption medial to its temporary counterpart. Normally, when the temporary tooth is lost, the erupting canine moves laterally and flares out to fit into the space between the upper canine and the upper lateral incisor. If a lower temporary canine is retained, its permanent replacement is forced to continue erupting medial to it. When partly erupted, the lower permanent canine will impinge on the hard palate, causing pain, inflammation, infection and, possibly, an oronasal fistula. This situation is exacerbated if the mandible is excessively narrow.

Upper canines

The upper permanent canines erupt rostral to their temporary counterparts. Retention of an upper temporary canine forces the perma-

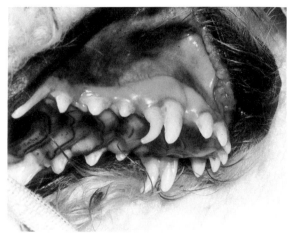

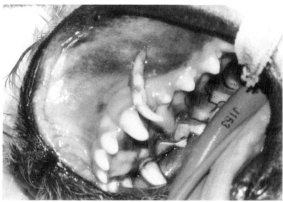

FIG. 1.7 Top: Retained temporary upper canine teeth, trapping debris and causing a localized gingivitis. Bottom: Extracted temporary upper canine tooth to show its position and size.

nent canine to erupt into the space intended for the opposing lower canine (Fig. 1.7). When the mouth is closed, the lower canine should close into the space between the upper canine and the upper lateral incisor. If that space is too small, the lower canine will collide with the erupting upper canine or the upper lateral incisor. This causes pain, which often induces excessive chewing and biting, and the following malocclusions:

- the upper or lower canine may be prevented from erupting fully, becoming impacted
- the lower canine may push the upper lateral incisor or the upper canine outwards
- the lower canine may be forced to erupt medial to the upper canine, impinging on the hard palate and possibly creating an oronasal fistula.

Incisors

The permanent incisors erupt caudal to their temporary counterparts. Retention of one or more incisors may interfere with the scissor occlusion, with upper incisors closing behind the lower incisors. This is not only important for 'showing', but may result in localized soft tissue trauma.

Extraction

Great care is required to loosen the retained temporary tooth without damaging the erupting permanent tooth. A sharp, fine elevator is carefully inserted between the tooth and gum and worked into the periodontal ligament round the two-thirds of the temporary tooth furthest away from the erupting tooth. Gradually, with small lateral excursions of the elevator tip, the periodontal ligament is cut, and the tooth loosens. The remaining ligamentous tissue is cut with the elevator until the tooth comes out. The use of dental forceps may result in root fracture, so great must be taken if they are employed.

A large fragment of temporary tooth root left in place will continue to deviate the erupting permanent tooth: it should be removed with careful use of the fine sharp elevator or a root tip pick. It may be necessary to raise a flap to expose the alveolar bone over the root, as described in Chapter 8. Take great care to avoid damage to the erupting tooth.

If a very small fragment of temporary tooth root is left in its socket, it may exfoliate or be resorbed. However, in some cases, it may cause inflammation or cyst formation in the bone. Thus an attempt should be made to remove retained root fragments, without damaging the erupting permanent tooth. If this is not possible, it may be necessary to leave this small fragment, in which case, radiographs should be taken 3 months later to check for complications.

It is better to spend an extra few minutes elevating the whole tooth gently and carefully than to spend a frustrating half hour attempting to retrieve a fractured root tip.

Dental Records

It is important to keep accurate records of dental treatments. There are numerous ways of recording such data, the simplest being based on diagrams. Useful features of such a chart include:

- occlusion and gingiva shown in lateral views
- individual teeth clearly identifiable
- right and left clearly marked

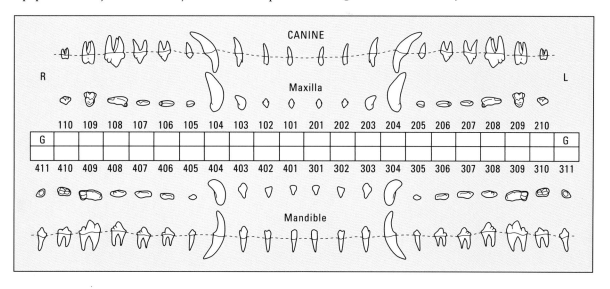

FIG. 1.8 A dental recording chart for dogs using the Modified Triadian System. (Reproduced by kind permission of Dentalabels.)

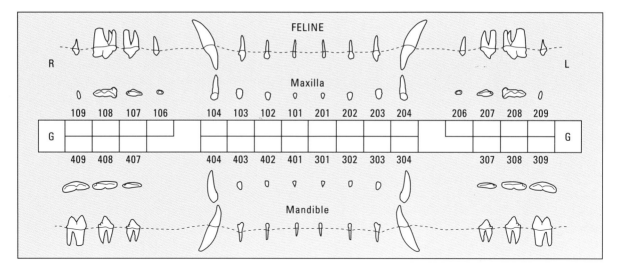

FIG. 1.9 A dental recording chaart for cats using the Modified Triadian System. (Reproduced by kind permission of Dentalabels.)

- specific spaces for annotation of precise disease details
- Space for details of the client, animal, relevant history and date are important for non-adhesive charts. Self-adhesive charts (Figs 1.8 and 1.9) are available that can be attached to patients' record cards.

Those shown here use the Modified Triadian System, where the first digit identifies the quadrant of permanent or temporary teeth (1–4 for permanent teeth, 5–8 for temporary teeth). The second and third digits refer to the location and anatomical description of the tooth. A tooth with the same anatomical designation should have the same identifying number, regardless of species. Gaps are left in the numbering system where there are missing teeth. Cats have only three upper premolars and two lower premolars. The missing first upper premolar and first and second lower premolars are left as gaps in the numbering system (see Fig. 1.9). The great advantages of this system are that it is unambiguous and can be entered on to computer records.

Other methods involve the annotation of teeth. They are numbered as seen from the front. For example, the right upper fourth premolar would be [4]PM and the left lower canine C[1]. Mistakes are easily made by putting the number in the wrong place, so care is required.

Structure of Teeth and Their Supporting Structures

Tooth Structure

Figures 1.10 and 1.11 show the internal structure of the canine and molar teeth. The bulk of the tooth's structure comprises dentine. The dentine of the crown, above gum level, is coated with enamel, whilst that of the root, below gum level, is coated with cementum. The fibres of the periodontal ligament are embedded in the cementum and the lamina dura of the alveolar socket, firmly attaching the tooth to the jaw.

Enamel

Enamel comprises 98% inorganic elements laid down in a hydroxyapatite lattice. It is insensitive and incapable of repair, although demineralized areas are capable of remineralization. An acellular membrane, the pellicle, covers the enamel. Plaque and calculus may adhere to this membrane. The enamel is contoured to form the enamel bulge near the gingival margin, which deflects food from the gingival crevice. This forms an important part of the natural defence mechanisms of the mouth and should be preserved. The enamel of

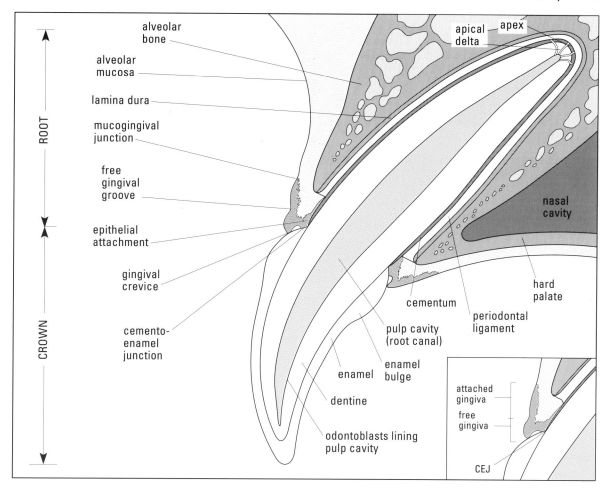

FIG. 1.10 Diagrammatic section through an upper canine of an adult dog.

dog and cat teeth is much thinner than that of humans. For clarity, the enamel in the diagrams of this book is drawn thicker than it really is.

Dentine

Dentine is organic, porous material, softer than enamel. It is capable of limited repair and responds to irritation and injury by producing layers of secondary dentine. More dentine is laid down continuously at the pulp margin by odontoblasts which line the pulp chamber, thickening the dentine wall, narrowing the pulp chamber and closing the apex. This process takes place at a rapid rate between the ages of 3 and 20 months, then proceeds at a much slower rate (Fig. 1.12). There are approximately 40,000 dentinal tubules radiating out from the pulp chamber through the dentine towards the enamel. These contain the apical processes of the odontoblasts and nerve endings, rendering the dentine a sensitive substance.

Cementum

Cementum is a type of bone which coats the dentine of the root. The periodontal ligament fibres are embedded in it and the lamina dura of the alveolus.

Cementoenamel junction

The cementoenamel junction is the junction between the crown and root of the tooth. The epithelial attachment of the gingiva joins gum to tooth here. As periodontal disease progresses, so this attachment migrates apically (towards the tip of the root).

Pulp

The pulp occupies the pulp cavity of the tooth. It comprises a matrix of odontoblasts and mesenchymal cells, with blood vessels, nerves and lymphatics which enter the tooth through the apex.

Apex

The apex of the tooth is the tip of the root. Unlike most human teeth, dog canine teeth usually have an apical delta: a few millimetres from the anatomical apex, the main pulp canal divides into a complexity of very narrow canals which radiate peripherally to the periodontium (Hennet, personal communication). Occasionally, a single canal forms the apex, as in the majority of humans. The morphology is probably similar for incisors, premolars and molars and for feline dentition, but the necessary research has not been completed.

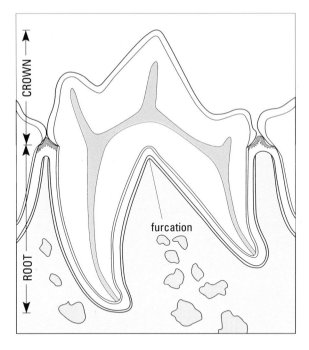

FIG. 1.11 Diagrammatic section through a lower first molar of an adult dog.

Development of Newly Erupted Permanent Teeth

At eruption, the dentine wall of the permenant tooth is thin, the pulp chamber is

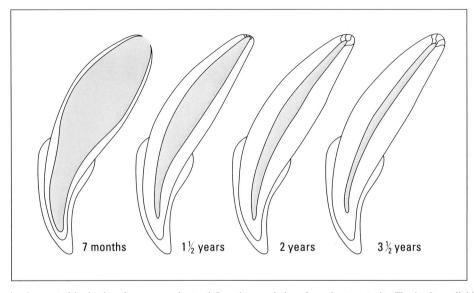

FIG. 1.12 The development of the dentine of an upper canine tooth from the completion of eruption to maturity. The dentine wall thickens, the pulp chamber becomes smaller and the apex closes to form the apical delta or the apical foramen. Adapted from H. Schmidt and P. Fahrenkrug, *Der praktische Tierarzt*, **5**, 16 (1987).

large and the apex is open. The newly erupted permanent tooth is thus a relatively weak structure, easily fractured. During the first 2 years, the odontoblasts continually produce new dentine, thickening the dentine wall and narrowing the pulp chamber. The apex gradually closes, forming the apical delta in the majority of dogs, or a very narrow single apical canal. The permanent teeth of a 2-year-old dog are therefore much stronger than those of a younger dog. The odontoblasts continue to lay down new dentine throughout life but at a much slower rate from 2 years old onwards. Reparative or secondary dentine is also produced by the odontoblasts in response to irritation or injury to the pulp (Fig. 1.13).

The Periodontium

The periodontal tissues, the supporting structures around the teeth, comprise the periodontal ligament, the alveolar bone and the gingiva.

Periodontal ligament

The periodontal ligament comprises mainly collagen and elastic fibres embedded in the cementum and lamina dura (cribriform plate of alveolar bone). It acts as a shock absorber, allowing a little movement during mastication but not enough to damage the apical blood supply. Like any ligament, it will repair, but very slowly.

Alveolar bone

The alveolar bone is that part of the maxilla or mandible forming the alveolar socket, housing the tooth root. Beneath its periosteum is a radiologically distinct line, the lamina dura, a useful measure of periodontal damage.

Gingiva

The gingiva is a tough, protective layer of cornified, stratified, squamous epithelium, firmly

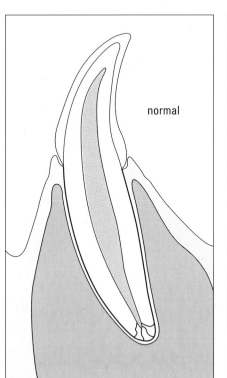
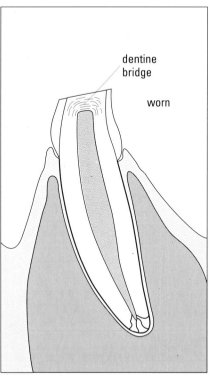

FIG. 1.13 The secondary dentine bridge produced to protect the pulp of a lower canine tooth suffering attrition. Left: Normal tooth. Right: Worn tooth with reparative dentine bridge.

bound to the underlying alveolar bone. It plays a major role in the defence against periodontal disease. It heals rapidly and is attached to the cementum near the cementoenamel junction by its epithelial attachment. The mucogingival line demarcates the junction between the alveolar mucosa and the attached gingiva (Fig. 1.14). The attached gingiva should be preserved at all costs: it is the dental surgeon's best friend.

Natural Defence Mechanisms of the Mouth

The aim of these defence mechanisms is to protect the teeth and the periodontium, particularly at the epithelial attachment of the gingiva.

Saliva

The saliva contains immunoglobulins (IgA) and a hydrogen peroxide-based antibacterial system. The salivary enzymes produce the peroxide. Potassium thiocyanate in the saliva is oxidized by hydrogen peroxide into hypothiocyanate, which is toxic to bacterial cells. This system is augmented by some enzymatic toothpastes and sprays.

Enamel bulge

The enamel bulge deflects anything being chewed from the free gingival margin, thus protecting the delicate epithelial attachment (Fig. 1.15).

Gingival crevice

The gingival crevice, or sulcus, lined by crevicular epithelium, is normally 1–3 mm deep. It allows a little movement of the free gingival margin without tearing the epithelial attachment and accumulates immunoglobulin-rich crevicular fluid.

Crevicular fluid

Crevicular fluid is produced by the tissue beneath the crevicular epithelium and diffuses through it into the gingival crevice. Saliva also accumulates here. This fluid is rich in immunoglobulins and other antibacterial agents, protecting the epithelial attachment and the underlying periodontal ligament from infection.

Attached gingiva

The attached gingiva is para-keratinized epi-

AM	alveolar mucosa
MGJ	mucogingival junction
AG	attached gingiva
IDF	interdental fold
FGG	free gingival groove
MG	marginal groove
IP	interdental papilla
FG	free gingiva

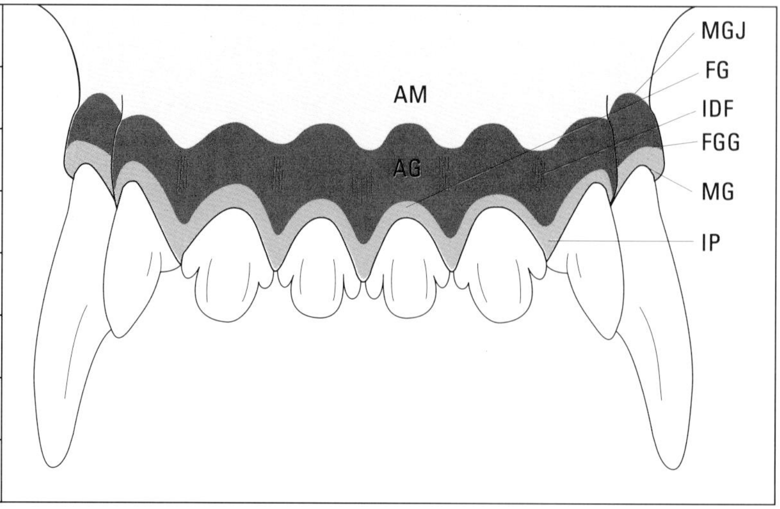

Fig. 1.14 The visible landmarks of clinically normal gingiva.

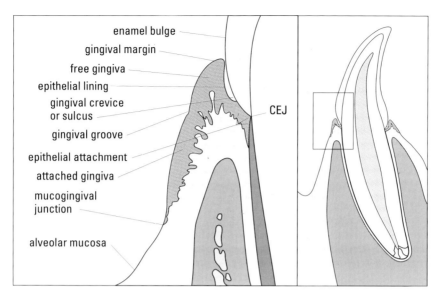

FIG. 1.15 The normal relationship between the gingiva and the tooth.

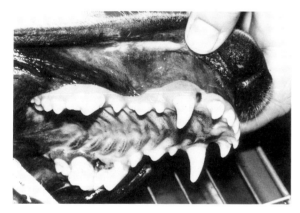

FIG. 1.16 The mucogingival line is clearly visible between the attached gingiva (non-pigmented in this dog) and the alveolar mucosa (pigmented in this dog).

thelium. It is much tougher tissue than the non-keratinized alveolar mucosa, which lies immediately beyond the mucogingival line. If the attached gingiva of a tooth is lost, the alveolar mucosa recedes rapidly and the tooth is lost. It is important to retain attached gingiva wherever possible.

All these defence mechanisms work together to protect the epithelial attachment under which lies the periodontal ligament. Great efforts should be made to retain as many of these features as possible in the mouth, to maximize its natural defences.

2
Hand Instruments

Hand Instruments

There are numerous dental hand instruments available. Each has: a handle, which may be solid or hollow; a shank, which is designed in various configurations; and a working tip. They are either double-ended, with two working tips, or single-ended. A basic set of hand instruments is listed below.

Hand instruments used primarily in periodontal treatment (Fig. 2.1):

- sickle-shaped supragingival scalers, e.g. SH 6/7
- subgingival curettes, e.g. SG 13/14
- Shepherd's crook explorer — often part of double-ended instrument, such as with a graduated periodontal probe, e.g. XP 23/QW
- graduated periodontal probe — the 1–3 mm graduations may be marked as indented lines, painted indented lines, or 1–3 mm painted blocks
- periosteal elevator, e.g. 9/8E.

Hand instruments used primarily in restorative work (Fig. 2.2):

- dental mirror, e.g. size 3
- dental spoon excavator, e.g. EXC 32L
- plastic filling instrument (PFI) — No. 1 is the most universally useful metal PFI, with a rounded packing tip at one end and a flat, paddle-shaped 'beaver-tail' at the other end; acrylic PFIs are also available
- ballpoint applicator
- mixing spatula, e.g. SPT 24 — made as metal or 'disposable' plastic instruments.

Hand instruments used primarily in endodontics:

- root canal plugger, e.g. RCP 1/3 - these are also available as 'finger pluggers', the working tip being approximately 25 mm long,

with a 10 mm 'handle'
- root canal spreader, e.g. RCS 3 (a single-ended spreader) - these can also be used as root canal explorers and are available as 'finger spreaders'.

Within one type of instrument (e.g. subgingival curettes), there are numerous subtle variations. It is wise to select the exact style of hand instrument from a tray of assorted instruments, as it is difficult to know how an instrument will feel in the hand from looking at a picture. Each operator will find which instruments feel best. It is advisable to start with a basic set of instruments: as you gain experience in dentistry and wish to expand your selection, you will be better able to choose the instruments you like.

Hand Positioning

Modified Pen Grasp

Hand instruments are generally held in a 'modified pen grasp' (Fig. 2.3). This provides maximum control of the instrument, precision, a wide range of movement, and good tactile sensation by the operator through the instrument.

The instrument is held between the tips of the thumb and the index finger, near the junction between the handle and the shank. These fingers do not touch each other, so the handle is visible between them. The handle rests against the hand somewhere between the thumb and the knuckles.

The middle finger is used to guide the instrument and to detect tactile sensations, for example, when the instrument's working tip contacts a rough surface. The pad of the finger, not the side, rests on the shank.

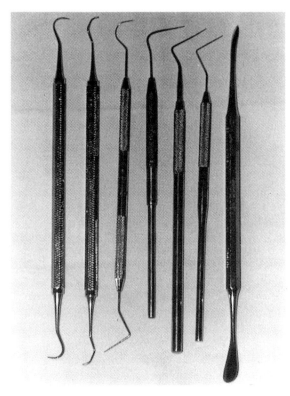

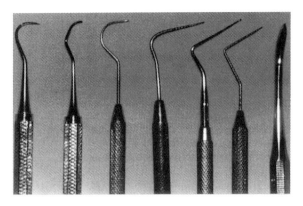

FIG. 2.1 Hand instruments used mainly for periodontal treatment, with detail of their working tips. From left to right: sickle-shaped supragingival scaler (SH 6/7); subgingival curette (SG 13/14); shepherd's crook explorer and graduated periodontal probe (XP 23/ QW); graduated periodontal probe with the 1–2 mm graduations marked as indented lines, painted indented lines, and painted blocks; periosteal elevator (9/8E).

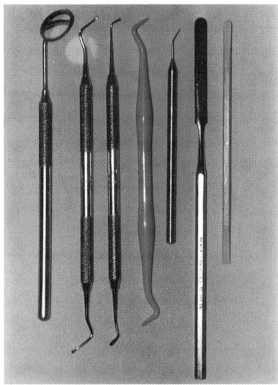

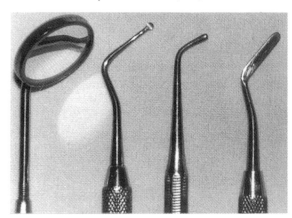

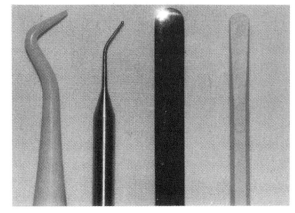

FIG. 2.2 Hand instruments used mainly for restorative work, with detail of their working tips. From left to right: dental mirror; dental spoon excavator (EXC 32L); plastic filling instrument (PFI) No. 1 (round end and beaver-tail end); acrylic PFI; ballpoint applicator; metal mixing spatula (SPT 24); 'disposable' plastic mixing spatula.

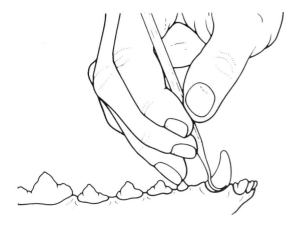

FIG. 2.3 The modified pen grip, using the fourth finger on the first premolar as a fulcrum to scale the lower canine with a supragingival scaler.

The index and middle fingers are bent, with the thumb bent outwards or held straight. These fingers should never be tense; a relaxed grasp is necessary to allow irregularities in the tooth surface to be felt.

Fulcrum

The pad of the fourth finger is used as a fulcrum. It is placed on a structure adjacent to the tooth to be worked on. This helps to support and stabilize the working hand. Ideally, a stable tooth, close to and in the same arch as the one to be worked on, is used. The pad of the fourth finger rests on the occlusal or incisal

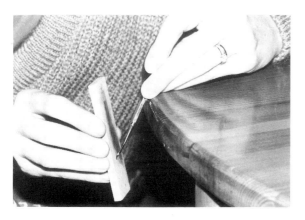

FIG. 2.4 Sharpening a supragingival scaler. Left: With a flat arcansas stone and oil. Right: With a conical arcansas stone and oil.

surface of the tooth. As the facial and lingual surfaces of the teeth tend to be coated in saliva, they are generally too slippery to use.

It is sometimes necessary to rest the fourth finger on the opposite arch, on the other hand, or on an object outside the mouth. Since the jaws are mobile, these are less secure than using an intraoral finger rest in the same arch.

Power-driven instruments are held in a pen grasp, using adjacent teeth as a fulcrum in the same way.

Sharpening Hand Instruments

Hand instruments with sharp edges need to be sharpened, preferably after each use, since the sharp edge is quickly lost. Attempting to work with blunt instruments is time-consuming and produces an unsatisfactory result. For example, curettage with a blunt curette tends to burnish plaque, calculus and

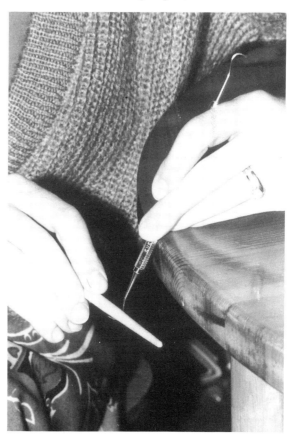

necrotic cementum onto the tooth, instead of scraping it off.

Procedure

There are numerous ways of sharpening instruments. The principle is to work the oiled sharpening stone against the instrument in a direction parallel with the machined surface, to remove a minute amount of metal.

A flat arcansas sharpening stone and some sharpening oil are used. A conical stone is also useful for instruments with small, curved, cutting edges, such as the dental spoon exavator. The instrument is held firmly, with the handle resting against the edge of a table and with the working tip protruding (Fig. 2.4). The sharpening stone is oiled. It is worked up and down against the machined edge of the instrument's working tip, starting at the heel (nearest the shank) and working round to the toe, ending with an upward stroke. The toe of a curette is rounded, so the stone is held at a flatter angle as it is worked round the toe, ending with an upward stroke. The technique is modified to suit each particular instrument.

Dental instrument sharpening kits are available with instructions through veterinary wholesalers.

If the working tip needs major sharpening, some dental instrument manufacturers provide such a service.

3
Power Equipment

Some form of power equipment is required to perform dentistry effectively. Teeth may be scaled using solely hand instruments, but power is required for polishing, which should be part of every dental prophylaxis. More advanced techniques involving the cutting of tooth structure necessitate power tools, as does mechanical scaling. The source of power which drives this equipment is either an electric engine or pressurized air. It is essential to cool the tooth with water or saline when using power equipment to avoid thermal damage to the pulp.

Mechanical Scalers

Electrical Ultrasonic Scalers

The scaling tip vibrates at 20–40 kHz in a longitudinal or elliptical direction. The cooling water is energized as it passes over the vibrating tip, providing it with scouring properties known as cavitation. This is not related to aerosol formation. Plaque, calculus, stains and debris are removed by the scaling tip and the cavitational activity of the water. A variety of scaling tips is available but the most useful is the sickle-shaped tip. The numerous ultrasonic instruments available fall into two categories:

Magnetostrictive vibration of the tip is caused by
(Fig. 3.1)   electromagnetic energy which changes the shape of the laminated ferromagnetic rod (the stack) inside the handpiece; the tip oscillates in an elliptical pattern.

Piezoelectric   changes in shape of the crystal within the handpiece cause the vibration of the tip, which oscillates in a linear pattern.

Both types oscillate in a longitudinal fashion, more complex designs exhibiting an elliptical movement. The piezoelectric scalers have a smaller handpiece than magnetostrictive scalers but, due to the brittle nature of the crystal, tend to be more easily damaged.

Air-Driven Scalers

Sonic Scalers

The scaling tip vibrates at less than 20 kHz (usually 16–20 kHz) with a more elliptical, longitudinal oscillatory pattern. The sonic scaler handpiece fits onto the high-speed air outlet of an air-driven dental unit. The cooling water flows over the vibrating tip, forming an aerosol and sometimes becoming energized enough to provide cavitation. If the scaler is pressed too hard on to the tooth (a load of over 100 g) the tip will not be able to vibrate, although the instrument will make the same sound. Several different scaling tips are produced, but the most useful is the sickle-shaped scaling tip (Fig. 3.2).

Rotosonic Scalers

A six-sided, non-cutting, 'roto-pro' bur is inserted in the high-speed handpiece and rotates at approximately 300,000 rpm. When held against a tooth, it shatters the surface, dislodging calculus, which is flushed away by the

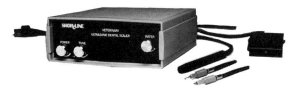

FIG. 3.1 Ultrasonic scaler.

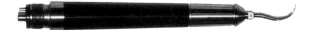

FIG. 3.2 Sonic scaler.

cooling water. As it is easy to damage enamel, dentine, pulp and soft tissues with these burs, they should not be used. Human patients complained of such dental pain after their teeth had been cleaned with rotosonic scalers that their use was abandoned by dentists. We should not subject our anaethetized animals to such unnecessary postoperative pain.

Although there are differences between sonic and ultrasonic scalers, the clinical response to both seems very similar. Rotosonic scalers are not used in human dentistry and should not be used in animal dentistry.

Mechanical Drill Units

Electric Engine-Driven Dental Units

These units are less expensive than air-driven units, but suffer several disadvantages (see Fig. 3.3). They are of low speed, rotating the bur at speeds of less than 90,000 rpm, so they tend to 'walk' off the tooth whilst drilling instead of cutting into it. There is no provision

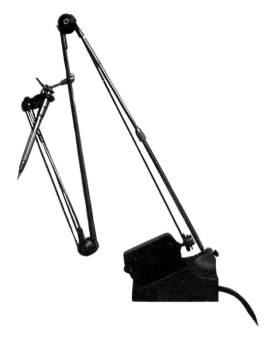

FIG. 3.4 Belt-driven dental unit.

RELATIVE ADVANTAGES (A) AND DISADVANTAGES (D) OF ELECTRICALLY AND AIR-DRIVEN DENTAL UNITS				
	Electrically driven dental units		Air-driven dental units	
Torque	high	A	low	D
Speed	low	D	low and high	A
Vibration	often	D	none	A
Use	awkward	D	easy and delicate	A
Heat	hot; needs irrigation	D	water-cooled high speed	A
Cost	lower	A	higher	D
Portability	usual	A	available	D
Handpieces and burs	limited range	D	huge choice	A
Handpieces	large, cumbersome	D	small, delicate	A

FIG. 3.3 Relative advantages (A) and disadvantages (D) of electrically and air-driven dental units.

for automatic water cooling of the bur, which heats up considerably during use; a constant flow of cooling water or saline on to the cutting end during operation is essential to prevent excessive heating of tooth structure or bone.

The dremel tool and the laboratory bench engine have many features in common. They take only a straight handpiece and use long-shanked straight handpiece burs and mandrels. This, combined with the size of the handpiece and the weight of the direct drive cable, make these units cumbersome in the confines of the mouth; manoeuvrability is restricted.

All these electrically driven units are rather clumsy relative to air-driven units. Their advantages are their high torque, low cost and portability. Several types are available.

Dremel tool

These are commonly used for model making. Sophisticated types are made for domiciliary dentistry. The engine is normally in the handpiece, and is powered by either a battery or, via an electric cable, the mains. Some have a direct-drive cable transmitting power from the engine to the handpiece, allowing the use of smaller handpieces. They can run at up to 30,000 rpm. These are the cheapest source of power.

Laboratory bench engine

Often used in dental laboratories, these engines are also used in human hospitals. They usually run at approximately 15,000 rpm, although some may reach 30,000 rpm. A direct-drive cable separates the engine from the handpiece.

Belt-driven dental unit

Until the 1950s, virtually all dental work was performed using the belt-driven unit (Fig. 3.4). It has a very low-speed (up to 20,000 rpm), high-torque engine, which generates much less heat to the handpiece than the dremel tool or the laboratory bench engine. Care must be taken to avoid tangling hair in the belt drive. It is more manoeuvrable than the dremel tool or the laboratory bench engine and can be used with both contra-angle and straight handpieces. These units are available second hand, so their prices vary.

Electric engine

These are often used for domiciliary work in the dental profession and sometimes solely as polishers (Fig. 3.5). Running at up to 90,000 rpm, they accept straight, contra-angle, prophy-angle and friction-grip handpieces. This im-

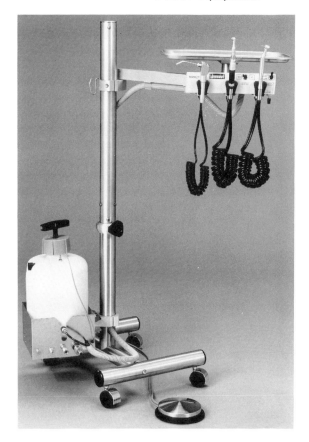

FIG. 3.6 Air-driven dental unit.

proves their manoeuvrability in the mouth. There is usually a micro-motor at the base of the handpiece which may heat up with extended continuous use. The motor may burn out after repeated stalling and water and oil contamination.

Prophymatic units have an oscillating head which produces less heat and avoids the problem of hair winding around the polisher head. Hence these units are longer lasting.

Electric scaler-polisher units

Electric units are available which combine an ultrasonic scaler and a low-speed drill unit. The low-speed drill accepts the straight, contra-angle, prophy-angle and friction-grip handpieces, making it a very useful, versatile piece of equipment.

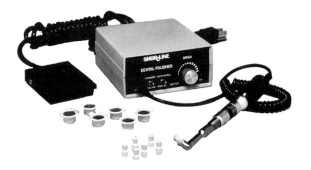

FIG. 3.5 Electric polisher unit.

Air-Driven Dental Units

Pressurized air from a compressor or a cylinder is used to turn an air turbine in the head of each handpiece at up to 400,000 rpm. At this speed the drill is much easier to control. It will cut through tooth structure quickly without 'walking' off the tooth. Air-driven units usually have both a high-speed and a low-speed handpiece (Fig. 3.7). The low-speed straight handpiece (up to 5000 rpm) accepts prophy-angle and contra-angle heads for use with polishing cups and friction-grip or latch-type attachments. The high-speed handpiece takes friction-grip burs and has a controllable water supply for cooling the cutting tip and flushing away debris. A fibreoptic light can be fitted in the high-speed handpiece to illuminate the cutting area. For cutting tooth structure, the high-speed handpiece is used at top speed (400,000 rpm), its most efficient, least damaging cutting speed. The disadvantages of air-driven dental units are their lack of torque and their high cost; however, air-driven units are easily the best to use, enabling the clinician to produce the best results with minimal difficulties.

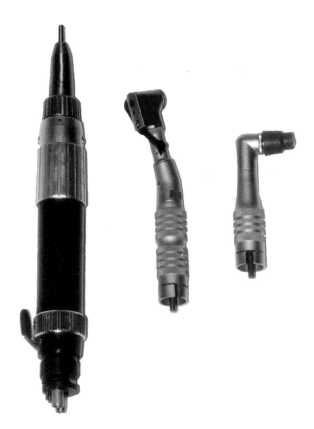

FIG. 3.8 Low-speed handpiece (straight handpiece) with a latch-type contra-angle attachment (centre) and a prophy-angle attachment (right).

Handpieces

There are several types of handpiece available (Fig. 3.7), each accepting various types of bur.

High-Speed Handpiece

This is exclusively an air-turbine handpiece for use on an air-driven dental unit at approximately 400,000 rpm. Burs are held in place by a friction-grip mechanism in the head, and hence are referred to as friction-grip burs. This combination optimizes efficiency and accuracy. A fibreoptic light can be fitted to the high-speed handpiece, to illuminate the area around the bur head.

Low-Speed Handpiece

This handpiece may be air or electrically driven. As part of the air-driven dental unit, it will run at up to 5000 rpm in forward or re-

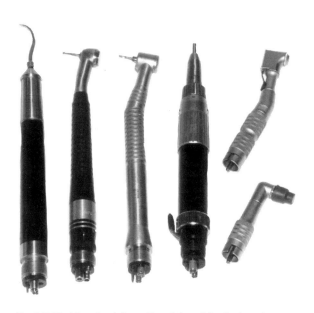

FIG. 3.7 Air-driven handpieces. From left to right: Sonic scaler, two high-speed handpieces, low-speed handpiece (straight handpiece), contra-angle attachment and prophy-angle attachment.

verse directions. When electrically driven, as there is no high-speed handpiece, the low-speed handpiece operates at speeds of up to 90,000 rpm, with a foot control or rotating knob to adjust the speed. Low-speed handpieces lack water cooling and so require a flow of saline over the operating tip. They are used in three forms (Fig. 3.8).

Straight handpiece

This is the low-speed handpiece unit. It accepts straight, long-shanked burs and mandrels. The burs are available as dental or surgical burs; the latter have two grooves around the shank, halfway up, to prevent blood from running up into the handpiece. Some of the dental burs are used for trimming acrylic. The mandrel takes sanding discs and diamond discs (to be used with great care and preferably not at all).

Contra-angle attachment

This fits onto the straight handpiece. As its name implies, it comprises two angles: a 25° angle and a 90° angle. It redirects the working tip to 65° to the horizontal, improving access to the many awkward areas of the mouth. Latch or friction-grip types are available. Being of low speed, its main uses are slow removal of dentine e.g. deep caries, finishing and sanding restorations, filling root canals using lentulo spirals and inserting small dental pins. Prophy heads are also available for polishing with the contra-angle.

Prophy-angle attachment

This attaches directly onto the straight handpiece and is used for polishing. A rubber prophy cup is fastened onto the button at 90° to the horizontal, at the operating end of the prophy-angle. Filled with prophy paste, the cup is rotated at up to 1000 rpm to polish teeth and certain restorations. Disposable prophy-angle attachments are also available. Prophy is short for dental prophylaxis, a term frequently misused to mean the scaling and polishing procedure.

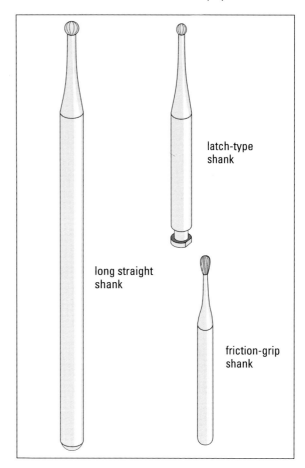

FIG. 3.9 Types of shank.

Burs

There are numerous styles of bur head mounted on three types of shank. The type of bur head chosen depends on the type of cut required, whilst the type of shank chosen depends on the handpiece to be used. Most bur styles are available on all types of shank.

Types of Shank

Long straight shank

The long straight shank (Fig. 3.9) fits directly into the straight low-speed handpiece. Usually, these burs are over 40 mm long. In dental catalogues, they are referred to as HP (for handpiece).

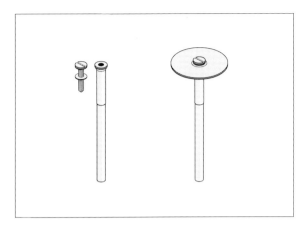

FIG. 3.10 Screw-top mandrel.

Latch-type shank

These shanks are designed to fit the latch-type handpiece which is often a contra-angle handpiece (Fig. 3.9). The bur is held in place by a latch in the handpiece which fits into a groove on the shank of the bur. This allows the bur a little lateral movement, causing it to wobble and introducing inaccuracies, which is why they are not used at high speed. They are usually about 20 mm long and are referred to in dental catalogues as RA (for right angle).

Friction-grip shank

This shank (Fig. 3.9) fits into friction-grip types of handpieces, which are the high-speed

and some contra-angle handpieces. They are usually approximately 20 mm long and are referred to in dental catalogues as FG (for friction grip).

Mandrels

There are HP, FG and RA types of mandrel. Diamond discs, sanding discs and polishing wheels and cups can be fitted onto the mandrel by screws (Fig. 3.10), push-on buttons and other methods.

Types of Bur Head

Bur heads are made of steel, stainless steel, tungsten carbide or steel coated in diamond grit of various grit sizes (coarseness). The most durable are tungsten carbide and diamond-coated. Burs are made with various head shapes, relating to their function (Fig. 3.11).

Pear

This is the most universally useful shape and also comes in a long size. This is the 330 series of burs. In ascending order of size, there are 329, 330, 331, 332, 333 and, with the longer head, 331 L, 332L, 333L: this is the US numbering system, other systems being variable. They are used for cutting enamel and dentine, cavity preparation, removing caries and creating undercuts adequate for the retention of fillings.

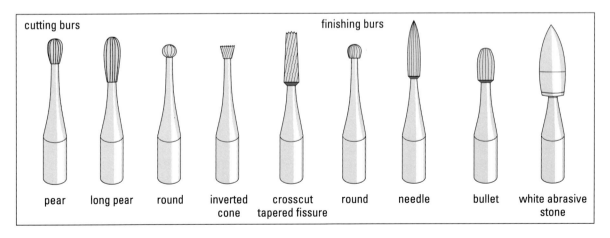

FIG. 3.11 Types of bur head

Round

This is a very useful shape, particularly for cavity preparation, cutting enamel and dentine and, with size $\frac{1}{2}$ creating undercuts as an alternative to inverted cone burs. Sizes run from $\frac{1}{2}$ to 9. The larger sizes are useful for removing caries in large cavities, safely, whilst the smaller sizes can be used to make access into root canals.

Fissure

Cross-cut or plain-cut, dome-ended, straight or tapered, these burs are particularly useful for sectioning multi-rooted teeth prior to extraction. They are far safer and easier to use than the diamond disc so often advertised for sectioning teeth. Sizes are 699, 700, 701, 702, 703, 700L, 701L for cross-cut tapered fissure burs and 169, 170, 171, 172 for plain-cut tapered fissure burs. Cross-cut burs are theoretically quicker at cutting, as debris is expelled from these burs more efficiently, minimizing clogging. Straight fissure burs are often used to drill into the cavity, to ensure that the enamel edges are vertical.

Inverted cone

These are used primarily to create undercuts for filling retention. It is generally thought that a small round or pear-shaped bur produces a better undercut, as rounded edges pack with filling material more efficiently than sharp angles. Sizes range from $33\frac{1}{2}$ to 37.

Finishing burs

These 12 to 40-bladed burs are used to shape and finish composite and amalgam. The most useful shapes of 12-bladed finishing burs are the 7901 series (needle-shaped), the 7404 (bullet-shaped) and the 7006 (round). An even better finish is obtained with 40-bladed burs, but it is advisable to produce the final finish of all restorations with finishing cups and discs, white stone, silicone rubber abrasive or finishing burs designed for final smoothing and polishing.

Abrasives

Green abrasives, made of silicone carbide grit, are used for the smooth grinding of enamel and finishing amalgam. White abrasives are made of fine white alundum grit and are used for finishing composite and glass-ionomer restorations.

4
Radiographic Techniques

Dental radiographs can be taken using veterinary or dental X-ray machines, screened or non-screened film, intra- or extraoral film positioning, and parallel or bisecting angle techniques. There are also several aids to developing the small dental films.

Radiographs are useful for many dental procedures, for purposes of diagnosis and verification. For example, during endodontic therapy, radiographs are taken: at the beginning of the procedure, to check the root canal; part way through the procedure, to ensure that the file reaches the apex; and after filling the root canal, to verify that there is an apical seal. If a vital pulpotomy is performed, radiographs are taken at the beginning and end of the procedure, as well as some months post-operatively, to monitor pulpal vitality and ensure that no complications have developed. Periodontal pockets, bone loss and apical abscesses can all be more accurately assessed radiographically, enabling the provision of more appropriate treatment (e.g. the extraction of the correct tooth).

X-Ray Units

Dental or manoeuvrable veterinary X-ray units can be used for both intra- and extraoral dental radiography. Fixed units are much more difficult to use. Second-hand dental X-ray units may be available from dentists, dental hospitals, dental wholesalers and dental journals, at reasonable prices.

Fixed-Head X-Ray Units

If it is not possible to alter the direction of the X-ray beam, foam wedges can be inserted under an extraoral X-ray plate to alter the angle of the film, and under the head to change the angle of the long axis of the tooth, for both intra- and extraoral radiography. When using bisecting angle techniques (see below), this moves the bisecting angle to a position at 90° to the X-ray beam. The same applies to parallel techniques (see below), as the parallel film and long axis of the tooth are moved to 90° to the X-ray beam.

Intraoral Radiography

Small, non-screened film is placed inside the mouth, adjacent to the particular tooth or quadrant to be radiographed. The X-rays are directed from outside the mouth, through the tooth to the film. This avoids the confusing superimposition of the image of the opposite arcade that is usually produced with extraoral radiography.

The hard palate of dogs and cats is flatter than that of man, necessitating the use of the bisecting angle technique when an intraoral technique is used to radiograph the maxillary cheek teeth. It is rarely preferable to use an extraoral parallel technique for these teeth. With smaller dogs and cats, it is sometimes a little awkward to position the films in their mouths. However, these are small inconveniences when compared with the clarity, accuracy and ease of interpretation of intraoral radiographs. Intraoral radiography is certainly an excellent technique for mandibular and maxillary diagnosis when teeth are involved.

X-Ray Film

Any type of X-ray film, screened or non-screened, can be used for intraoral radiography. However, the use of the smaller, non-screened, dental X-ray film allows accurate, clear radiographs to be taken with ease. The sizes of most use for veterinary dentistry are 'occlusal' at 54 x 70 mm and 'standard' at 30 x 40 mm. If duplicate copies of a radiograph are required, a double film packet is used, containing two separate films. There are numerous manufacturers of non-screened dental X-ray film, but they can be categorized according to their developing technique

Instant, self-developing, non-screened, dental film

This involves the injection of developer into the film envelope, either from a special bottle (Fig. 4.1) or syringe or, by pulling a tab, from a seperate compartment of the film envelope. The film is developed in 15 to 60 seconds; the envelope is then opened under running water, and the film rinsed and ready for inspection.

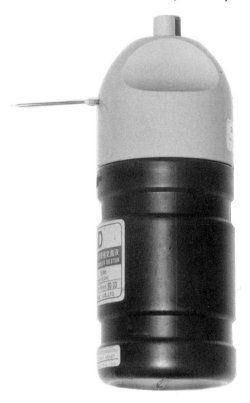

FIG. 4.1 The Hanschin pusher system for the injection of the developer–fixer solution into the film envelope is very similar to the Prestige pusher system.

This is not an expensive system, particularly considering its great convenience.

The box containing non-screened dental intraoral film usually carries details of recommended exposures and focal lengths for that particular type of film, when using a dental X-ray unit. The most satisfactory focal length using a veterinary X-ray unit is usually 20 cm; any less than this may result in inaccuracies from the divergence of the beam. As there is often some variation between X-ray machines, it is difficult to state exact exposures, but the following exposures, for a focal length of 20 cm, can be taken as guidelines for use with non-screened intraoral film:

Small dogs, and cats	60–70 kVp 20 mA 0.5–0.8 seconds	
Medium and large dogs	70–80 kVp 20 mA 0.8–1.0 seconds	

It is wise to experiment with your own X-ray machine and a skull to determine the optimal exposures. A paper clip is useful to assess any magnification or distortion of the image: the paper clip is placed on the tooth, the radiograph taken and developed and the paper clip then laid on top of its image for comparison.

Ordinary non-screened film

This type of film is developed using an automatic processor, a series of darkroom tanks with a multiple-clip dental X-ray film holder, or a chairside lightsafe box of mini-processing jars (Fig. 4.2) with a single-clip dental X-ray film holder. The film is developed in 2–6 minutes.

Techniques

The technique used is dictated by the teeth to be radiographed. The parallel technique is employed when radiographing the lower premolars and molars. The bisecting–angle technique is used to accommodate the length of the canine root and the flatness of the hard palate, in producing an accurate radiograph of the maxillary teeth and the mandibular incisors and canines. Maxillary cheek teeth can also be radiographed using an extraoral parallel technique.

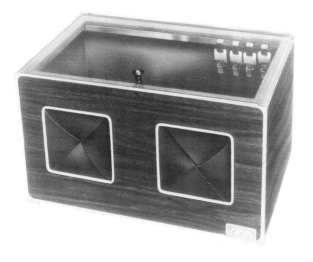

Parallel technique

To minimize any distortion of the shape or size of the image when using this technique, the film must be as close as possible to the tooth and absolutely parallel to its long axis.

The animal is positioned in lateral recumbency with the side to be radiographed uppermost. The intraoral film is placed lingual (medial) to the lower premolars or molars to be radiographed, with the sensitive side towards the X-ray tube. It is pushed ventrally so that its most ventral edge is level with the inferior border of the mandible. The film is also pressed against the tooth and mandible. Thus the film is parallel with the long axis of the tooth and is as close as possible to the tooth. It is held in this position by foam wedges, cotton wool or crumpled paper towels. The X-ray beam is directed at 90° to the film and the parallel long axis of the tooth (Fig. 4.3).

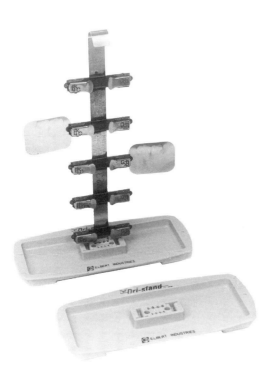

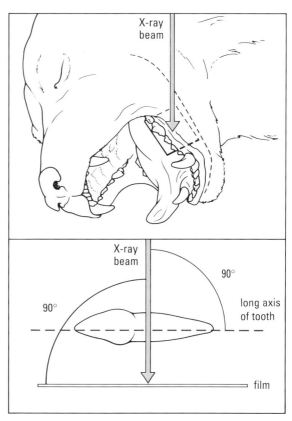

FIG. 4.2 Top: A chairside dental film developing system of mini-processing jars containing developer, water, fixer, then water, with clips for handling the films. Bottom: A drip-stand for drying the radiographs.

FIG. 4.3 Parallel technique for intraoral radiography.

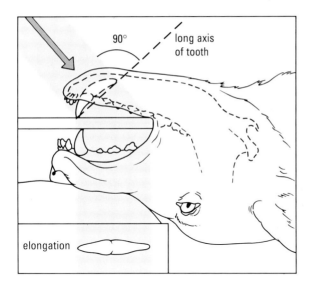

Fig. 4.4 Directing the X-ray beam at right angles to the long axis of the tooth, elongating the tooth's image.

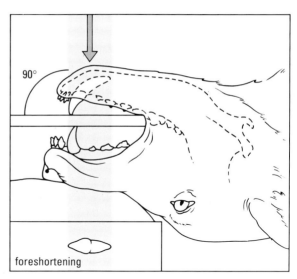

Fig. 4.5 Directing the X-ray beam at right angles to the film, shortening the tooth's image.

Bisecting-angle technique

This technique was devised to overcome the difficulties of obtaining accurate images of the teeth imposed by the shapes of the teeth and their surrounding structures. In the confines of the mouth it is often impossible to place a film close and parallel to the long axis of a tooth. If the beam is then directed at 90° to the long axis of the tooth, the image will be elongated (Fig. 4.4). Similarly, if the beam is directed at 90° to the film, the image will be foreshortened (Fig. 4.5). If a line is drawn between the long axis of the tooth and the film, bisecting the angle between the two, and the X-ray beam is directed at 90° to this line, the image will be neither elongated nor foreshortened, but an accurate representation of the tooth (Fig. 4.6). This is the principle of the bisecting-angle technique, the method of choice for producing accurate radiographs of the incisor and canine teeth, and some maxillary cheek teeth.

The animal is placed in sternal recumbency for radiography of the maxillary incisors, canines, premolars and molars, and dorsal recumbency for radiography of the mandibular canines and incisors. The long axis of a tooth approximates to a line drawn between the apex and the tip of the crown. The apex of the

canine tooth is level with the rostral root of the second premolar.

The film is placed in the mouth on the occlusal surfaces of the teeth. When non-screened dental X-ray film is used, it can be angled towards the long axis of the tooth, bringing the film both closer and more parallel to the tooth (Fig. 4.7). This is of particular help when radiographing the canines. It is essential

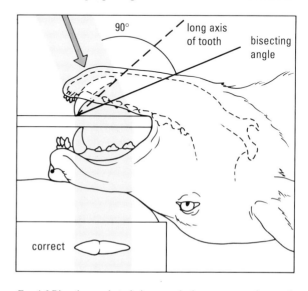

Fig. 4.6 Bisecting-angle technique, producing an accurate image of the tooth.

that the film is not bent, as this will distort the image.

The bisecting angle is visualized and the X-ray beam directed at 90° to it. The film position is checked, to ensure that the apex will not miss the film. When radiographing the canines and incisors, the beam is directed obliquely rostro-caudally, whereas for the cheek teeth, the beam is directed latero-medially.

In the mesaticephalic breeds, the bisecting angle for the maxillary canine approximates to a line between the tip of the crown and the centre of the eye, when the X-ray plate is inside the mouth and parallel with the hard palate.

Extraoral Radiography

Small dental film, larger non-screened film or screened film may be used for extraoral radiography. With the exception of the parallel technique employed to radiograph the maxillary cheek teeth, extraoral radiography produces some degree of superimposition of the opposing arcade, creating a rather confusing picture.

Techniques

Parallel technique

The maxillary molars and premolars can be radiographed accurately without the superimposition of the opposite arcade using this extraoral technique. The animal is placed in dorso-lateral recumbency with the side to be radiographed nearest the table. The mouth is opened as wide as possible and the head is tilted until the long axis of the maxillary tooth is parallel with the table. The film is placed on the table immediately underneath the tooth. The X-ray beam is directed at 90° to the film (Fig. 4.8). The opposite arcade is just out of the field of view. It is the divergence of the cheek teeth and the width of the maxilla which allow this technique to succeed.

The mandibular cheek teeth of animals with a wide lower jaw can also be radiographed in this way.

Oblique lateral technique

Mandibular and maxillary cheek teeth can be radiographed using the oblique lateral technique. The superimposition of the opposing arcade and the foreshortening of the image usually complicate the interpretation of these radiographs.

The animal is placed in lateral recumbency with the X-ray plate under its head. The quadrant to be radiographed is placed on the X-ray plate. The mouth is held open with a radiolucent foam cylinder or mouth-gag. A

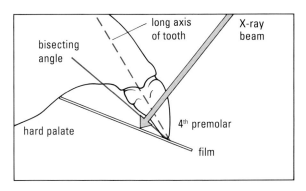

FIG. 4.7 Dental X-ray film angled towards the long axis of the upper fourth premolar, without bending the film or missing the apex.

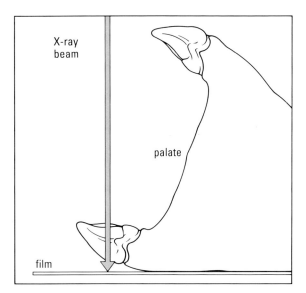

FIG. 4.8 Extraoral parallel technique for radiography of the upper premolars.

radiolucent triangular foam edge is used to tilt the head at 45°, raising the unwanted quadrants from the plate. The X-ray beam is directed at 90° to the plate (Fig. 4.9).

From the earlier section describing the bisecting-angle technique for intraoral rediography, it will be clear that the oblique lateral technique causes a degree of foreshortening of the image. The technique can easily be modified to overcome this problem, as follows.

Bisecting-angle technique

The animal and X-ray plate are arranged as for the oblique lateral technique. The average long axis of the teeth is visualized. A line bisecting the angle between the average long axis of the teeth and the X-ray film is then visualized. The X-ray beam is directed at 90° to the line of this bisecting angle.

Although the problem of foreshortening is thus overcome, the superimposition of the opposing arcade and other structures is still a complicating factor. The other techniques described earlier are easier to use.

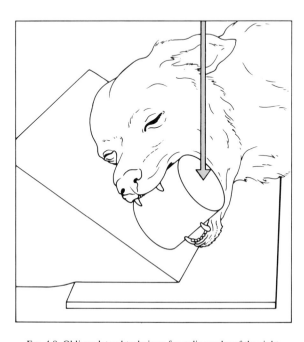

Fɪɢ. 4.9 Oblique lateral technique for radiography of the right mandibular premolars.

Summary of Techniques

For most situations, the following radiographic techniques are suggested.

Radiographic technique	Teeth to be radiographed
Intraoral bisecting angle	Maxillary and mandibular incisors and canines
Intraoral parallel	Mandibular premolars and molars
Extraoral parallel or intraoral bisecting angle	Maxillary premolars and molars

Interpretation of Dental Radiographs

Radiographs produced without distortion are of great use in dentistry and are far easier to interpret than those with superimposed, foreshortened or elongated images. Whole books have been devoted to this very involved subject, but only the most pertinent points will be broached here.

Lamina dura

When visible, the uninterrupted lamina dura suggests periodontal health (Fig. 4.10). A break in its path implies some periodontal pathology, but it is not pathognomonic. If the lamina dura is not visible radiographically, it does not necessarily mean that it is not there.

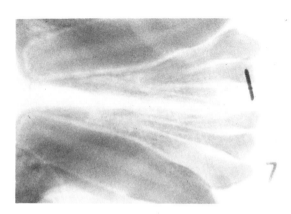

Fɪɢ. 4.10 Radiograph showing the lamina dura of the incisors and canines.

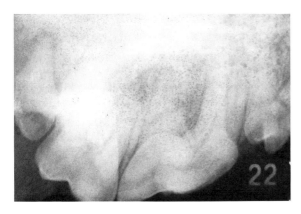

FIG. 4.11 Radiograph showing apical rarefaction of the caudal root of the upper fourth premolar.

Apical rarefaction

An 'apical halo' (Fig. 4.11) suggests several possible conditions:

- endodontic involvement, with pulpal pathology extending into the periapical bone; this may appear some months after pulpal pathology began or a conventional root canal treatment failed
- periodontal disease, when infection has tracked to the apex through the periodontal tissues; there will usually be additional evidence of periodontal disease, e.g. horizontal or vertical bone loss, lamina dura involvement and clinical evidence
- combination of periodontal and endodontic pathology where infection has reached the apex by both routes
- an apical cyst, which appears as an encapsulated radiolucency (rare in animals)
- normal feature.

Not all apical rarefaction is pathological in dogs and cats. Comparison should always be made with other teeth of the same type in the same animal. The periapical bone of the canine teeth of normal dogs often appears radiolucent. A distinctly round radiolucent area, however, is usually pathological.

Bone resorption

The degree of periodontal disease can be more accurately assessed with the aid of radiography.

Horizontal bone loss with suprabony pockets or without pockets, and vertical bone loss with infrabony pockets are easily visible. Once accurately diagnosed, appropriate treatment can be provided.

Fractures

Before any endodontic treatment is instigated, radiographs should be taken to ensure that the correct procedure is used. A fractured tooth root is one factor which must be detected, as the proposed course of action may need to be revised. Mandibular fractures are often associated with tooth roots, either as a result of trauma or an extension of severe periodontal or endodontic disease.

Buried root tips

Roots are frequently left in their alveolar sockets after the fracturing and loss of the crown, particularly in cats. This may be the result of trauma, the erosion of feline subgingival resorptive lesions or indelicate attempted extraction. Radiology is invaluable in the detection and location of these otherwise invisible roots which can be seen as more radiodense areas within the alveolar bone.

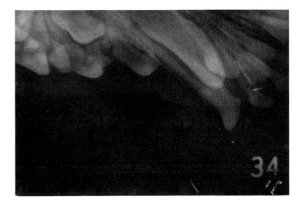

FIG. 4.12 Radiograph showing the presence of a full set of unerupted, permanent teeth beneath a full set of retained temporary teeth in a 6 month old Yorkshire Terrier.

Caries and Feline Subgingival Resorptive Lesions

Teeth with carious decay or resorptive lesions must be radiographed to determine the extent of the lesion. This will assist the selection of the appropriate treatment. Definitive diagnosis of resorptive lesions depends on radiography as much of each lesion is below the gingival margin. A post-operative radiograph is useful, to check for adequate filling.

Detection of Unerupted or Missing Permanent Teeth

If the permanent teeth have not erupted as expected, a series of radiographs will reveal the presence of any unerupted teeth (Fig. 4.12). Missing permanent teeth, a disqualification in 'showing', can be detected before the eruption of the permanent dentition has begun. This can be of great assistance in breeding and 'showing' situations.

5

Periodontal Disease, Therapy and Minor Periodontal Surgery

Periodontal Disease

Periodontal disease is a disease of the supporting structures of the teeth, the periodontium, which comprises the gingivae, the periodontal ligament and the alveolar bone. Over 87% of dogs and cats more than 3 years old have periodontal disease to a degree which would benefit from treatment. More teeth are lost as a result of periodontal disease than for any other reason; most of these teeth are healthy.

Aetiology

Plaque is the major cause of periodontal disease. It is composed of bacteria in a matrix of salivary glycoproteins and extracellular polysaccharides. The bacteria adhere to the pellicle, the acellular layer covering the exposed surfaces of all teeth. The plaque matrix then accumulates on this base. Plaque cannot be rinsed off. It has to be removed mechanically, with a toothbrush or, under anaesthetic, with dental scalers. If allowed to accumulate, plaque may become mineralized to form calculus. This is particularly common on the upper carnassial tooth, which is adjacent to the opening of the parotid duct, as saliva, the main source of these minerals, is deposited directly onto this tooth. Calculus alone is not pathogenic, but its rough surface is ideal for the retention of further plaque.

Predisposing Factors

A normal healthy mouth has approximately 750 million bacteria per millilitre of saliva.

The oral defence mechanisms maintain an equilibrium between these bacteria and the health of the tissues. This equilibrium shifts in favour of the bacteria when the oral defences are impeded. The major factors predisposing to periodontal disease interfere with these defences and include:

- overcrowded and rotated teeth, commonly seen in brachycephalic breeds
- retained temporary teeth, with plaque accumulating between the temporary and erupting permanent teeth
- a diet of entirely sticky food, with no tooth cleaning regime
- slab fractures of teeth, exposing rough dentine on which plaque accumulates (the loss of the enamel bulge exacerbates the situation)
- malocclusions
- trauma
- chemical irritants
- many systemic diseases
- reduced production or flow of saliva e.g. open-mouthed breathing, which dehydrates the saliva, impeding its defensive ability.

Pathogenesis

Initially, the bacteria in the supragingival plaque are the relatively non-motile, aerobic, Gram-positive cocci and rods. These irritate the gingivae, producing the first stage of periodontal disease, a marginal gingivitis, which is seen as a reddened line along the gingival margin. Gingivitis is reversible. A daily regime of effective tooth brushing should eliminate this early stage of gingivitis. If this marginal gingivitis is

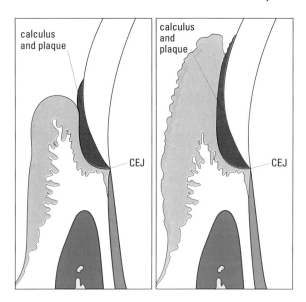

Fig. 5.1 Gingivitis. Left: Marginal gingivitis with gingival oedema and debris accumulating in the gingival pocket. Right: Gingival hyperplasia forming a 'false' gingival pocket.

not treated, the gingival margin becomes oedematous, opening up the gingival crevice and allowing easy access for the bacteria. Subgingival plaque begins to form, creating a gingival pocket (Fig. 5.1). The production of immunoglobulin-rich crevicular fluid increases. Inflammation increases and the gingivitis becomes more generalized, the gingiva often bleeding when touched. This stage is easily treated with a thorough scale and polish, followed by daily homecare. Without the homecare the situation rapidly deteriorates and within two months the mouth will be as bad as before.

Gingival hyperplasia or epulis is a common finding, particularly in Spaniels and Boxers. It may be a response to the presence of plaque, but it is usually thought to be of spontaneous or hereditary origin. It is often described as a benign fibrous tumour of the gingiva. The attached gingiva grows in an uncontrolled way to produce cauliflower-like gingival tissue on the facial surfaces of the gums, extending coronally towards the tips of the tooth crowns. This commonly covers the incisors and first premolars. These 'false' gingival pockets (Fig. 5.1) trap plaque and debris, encouraging the onset of periodontitis.

Untreated, the reversible gingivitis progresses to irreversible periodontitis. This deterioration may occur within weeks of the onset of gingivitis, or it may be several years before periodontitis develops. As the supra- and subgingival plaque accumulates, its bacterial flora changes to more tissue-destructive, motile, anaerobic, Gram-negative rods and filamentous organisms. Their endotoxins and the tissue response result in rapid progression of the disease (Fig. 5.2). As the plaque advances subgingivally, so the epithelial attachment migrates apically. If the gingival margin also recedes, the tooth root will be visibly exposed, coated in a layer of plaque and calculus, without the formation of a pocket. Usually, the gingival margin does not recede as fast as its epithelial attachment. Once the epithelial attachment has receded apically beyond the cementoenamel junction, a periodontal pocket has formed.

Alveolar bone and periodontal ligament are also destroyed by the inflammation. If the full thickness of the bone is destroyed, it is known as horizontal bone loss. In this case, the level of the receding epithelial attachment usually

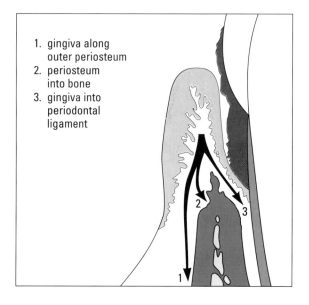

Fig. 5.2 Spread of endotoxins in periodontal disease. 1: through the gingiva and along the outer periosteum; 2: through the periosteum into the bone; 3: through the gingiva and into the periodontal ligament.

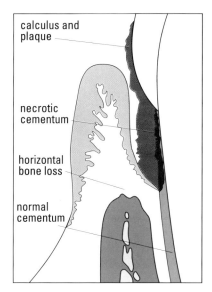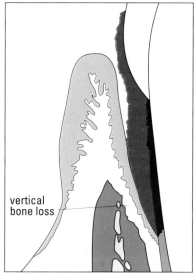

Fig. 5.3 Periodontal pockets. Left: Suprabony pocket. Right: Infrabony pocket.

remains of coronal to the crest of the bone, forming a suprabony pocket (Fig. 5.3). Sometimes, particularly around the incisors and premolars, the gingival margin recedes with its epithelial attachment and the alveolar bone, so no pocket forms. This is referred to as periodontitis without pocket formation. Around the molar and premolar teeth, the bone is often partially eroded. This bony destruction involving part of the thickness of the alveolar

bone is called vertical bone loss. The epithelial attachment commonly recedes apically beyond the crest of the alveolar bone, forming an infrabony pocket (Fig. 5.3). The endotoxins and inflammation produced by the bacteria in this pocket continue this vertical bone destruction, rapidly creating deep pockets, which usually exude pus.

Once over 50% of the periodontium has been destroyed, the tooth becomes mobile. The increased movement of the tooth weakens the remaining periodontal ligament. The bacterial attack continues, destroying more periodontal tissue, until finally the tooth is exfoliated. Most of the bacteria and debris are lost with the tooth, so the socket heals rapidly. Usually, after 3-6 months, the bone will regenerate to fill the socket.

Clinical Signs

The first stages of periodontal disease often exist without symptoms. A diagnosis depends on clinical examination. As the disease progresses, some clinical signs may develop. These vary from the purely oral signs of halitosis, dysphagia, excessive salivation, oral discomfort and haemorrhage, to a more generalized malaise. There may be evidence of associated disease in other organs, infected by the haematogenous spread of bacteria from the reservoir of infection in the mouth. The heart, kidneys and liver are commonly involved in this way.

Periodontal Therapy

The most important part of the treatment of periodontal disease is the through scaling and polishing of the teeth. Some degree of periodontal surgery is often required in addition, but there is no point in doing such surgery if the source of the problem, plaque, remains. Plaque and all other debris must be removed from the teeth, both above and below the gingival margin, in an effort to stop the progression of periodontal disease. The tooth sur-

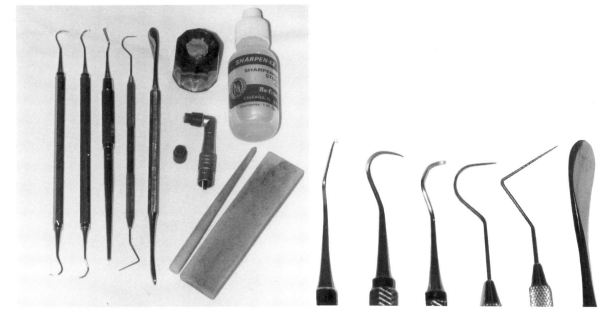

Fig. 5.4 Hand instruments and polisher used during a dental scale and polish. Left, from left to right: sickle-shaped supragingival scaler (SH6/7); subgingival curette (SG13/14); hoe (9MC); Shepherd's crook explorer with a graduated periodontal probe at the other end (XP23/Q W); periosteal elevator (9/8E); prophy paste in a dappen dish with the prophy-angle polishing head and a soft rubber prophy cup below; conical and flat arcansas sharpening stones with sharpening stone oil above. Right: Close-up of the heads of the hand instruments. From left to right: hoe; sickle-shaped supragingival scaler; subgingival curette; Shepherd's crook explorer; graduated periodontal probe; periosteal elevator.

faces must then be restored to their natural perfect smoothness, to deter the adherence of further plaque. Following all dental treatment, a homecare regime should be introduced to maintain good oral hygiene and to control or prevent the recurrence of periodontal disease.

Instrumentation

The equipment required to perform a scale and polish is as follows:

Rongeurs:	dental forceps, to crack off gross calculus deposits
Mechanical scalers:	ultrasonic or sonic scaler
Hand scalers and curettes:	the sickle-shaped supragingival scaler and the subgingival curette are the most useful
Sharpening stone and oil:	to sharpen the hand instruments daily; blunt instruments are worse than useless
Shepherd's crook explorer:	to detect subgingival calculus and cavities
Periodontal probe:	to measure pocket depth; it is usually part of a double-ended instrument, with the explorer at the other end
Scalpel blade:	for minor periodontal surgery
Polishing unit:	soft rubber prophy cup; prophy paste (preferably with fluoride) dispensed into a dappen dish, to avoid contamination of the remaining paste.
20 – 60 ml syringe:	containing dilute (0.1–2%) chlorhexidine or povidone-iodine with a bluntened 21 G needle: to flush debris from the gingival crevice.

Instrumentation is covered more fully in Chapters 2 and 3.

Scaling

Scaling is most effectively performed using a combination of ultrasonic or sonic scalers and hand scalers. Do not rely on mechanical scaling alone; it cannot do a thorough job. Scaling can be performed entirely using hand instruments. It may take a little longer but the end result should be very good.

Procedure

1. Gross calculus deposits are easily removed using a pair of rongeurs. Being careful to avoid damaging the gingivae, the rongeurs are closed across the calculus, which breaks and drops from the tooth.
2. A sickle-shaped supragingival scaler is used to pull the remaining, visible calculus off the crowns of the teeth always pulling away from the gingivae (Fig. 5.5).
3. The ultrasonic or sonic scaler is used to remove the residual plaque, calculus and debris. A plentiful water flow is essential to cool the oscillating tip and flush away the debris. When the frequency of oscillation and the water flow are correctly adjusted, an aerosol of water will form around the

oscillating tip. Gentle stroking of the tooth with the side of the sickle-shaped scaling tip seems to be the most effective and least damaging method of mechanical scaling (Fig. 5.6). If the scaling tip is pressed on to the tooth, it will not be able to oscillate properly, rendering it ineffective at debris removal; it will also create heat which causes inflammation and necrosis of the dental pulp, necessitating endodontic treatment and it will damage the tooth surface. Such iatrogenic damage also results from using the point of the scaler instead of the side, or holding it in one place; it should be moved continuously over the tooth surface, always moving away from the gingivae. In general, 15 seconds of continuous scaling is the maximum for any one tooth. If the tooth is not clean in that time, return to it in a minute, having scaled a few other teeth in the meantime. This will minimize iatrogenic damage.

Ultrasonic, sonic and rotosonic scalers are designed for use above the gingival margin. Once inserted into the gingival crevice or a pocket, the cooling water can no longer reach the oscillating tip, which rapidly does thermal damage to both hard and soft tissues. Subgingival excursions lasting half a second are permissible and may aid the removal of subgingival debris. The use of hand instruments for subgingival work is

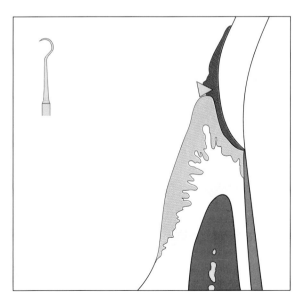

Fig. 5.5 Removing supragingival calculus with a supragingival scaler.

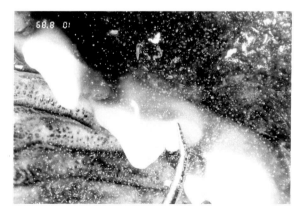

Fig. 5.6 Removing supragingival debris with a sonic scaler; note the water spray.

preferable. If the gingiva is carefully held
away from the tooth to allow the cooling
water to reach the tip and to flush out the
debris, mechanical scalers may be used
subgingivally. There are ultrasonic scalers
with hollow tips where the water comes out
of the end of the tip. These are designed
for use subgingivally as they irrigate the
subgingival area at the same time as removing plaque and calculus.

Exploration

Exploration with the tip of the shepherd's
crook explorer will identify any remaining
debris and erosive lesions of the tooth surface
(e.g. feline subgingival resorptive lesions). The
explorer skips on reaching any roughness of the
surface. The remaining debris can then be
removed and the tooth surface irregularities
treated.

Pocket Depth Measurement

Pocket depth measurement, using the graduated periodontal probe, will reveal any pockets
in need of periodontal surgery. The probe is
inserted into the gingival crevice until a firm,
soft resistance is felt. It is then moved around
the tooth with its blunt end running along the
epithelial attachment at the bottom of the crevice or pocket. The depth is easily measured
where the gingival margin meets the probe
(Fig. 5.7). The process is repeated around all
the teeth.

Pockets deeper than 4 mm may be normal,
but should be observed for signs of developing
periodontal disease. An inflamed pocket more
than 4 mm deep is difficult to keep clean;
debris will soon accumulate in the pocket and
periodontal disease may continue unabated.
Such 'pathological' pockets may need surgical
intervention. It is quite common to find a
normal gingival crevice 4–6 mm deep, particularly over the upper canines. If there are no
pathological changes present, it is not necessary
to perform gingival surgery. The uninflamed
gingiva will be closely applied to the tooth's

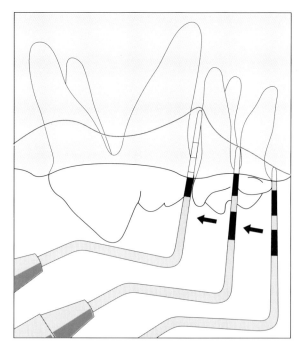

Fig. 5.7 Using the graduated periodontal probe to measure pocket
depth around the upper first molar and the upper fourth premolar.

surface, so debris is unlikely to accumulate in
the sulcus. The depth should be noted and the
gingivae examined every 6 months, looking for
signs of gingivitis. Only when it is apparent that
the oral defence mechanisms are failing is it
necessary to intervene surgically.

Subgingival Curettage

Subgingival curettage, the most important
step in the scale and polish, is the removal of
plaque, calculus, debris and excessive inflammatory epithelium from the gingival crevices and
pockets and the smoothing of any affected root
tissue (root planing), using a subgingival curette. Being curved in cross section, this instrument should not damage the gingivae when
used subgingivally.

Where the pockets are less than 4 mm deep,
closed curettage is usually employed. The curette is inserted into the gingival crevice with
its curved side against the gingiva and its sharp
edges towards the tooth, at an oblique angle,
with the toe (tip) of the curette pointing

apically. When soft but firm resistance is felt, at the bottom of the gingival crevice or pocket, the curette handle is tilted away from the tooth, engaging one sharp edge in the debris and cementum and the other sharp edge in the crevicular epithelium (Fig. 5.8). The instrument is then pulled towards the crown and out of the gingival crevice. This removes any debris from the tooth's surface and scrapes the crevicular epithelium, removing inflammatory, necrotic and oedematous tissue. Normal, smooth crevicular epithelium will not engage the edge of the curette and so should not be damaged. The process is repeated around each tooth with overlapping strokes.

A dental hoe can be used to remove subgingival debris (Fig. 5.9), but the crevicular epithelium is not scraped clean.

Any debris remaining in the gingival crevice or pockets will continue the course of periodontal disease as if the dental prophylaxis had never been performed; its removal is essential. When the root surface is involved, it should be thoroughly cleaned by 'root planing' (see Fig. 5.10). If the surfaces cannot be properly cleaned using closed curettage (e.g. if pocket

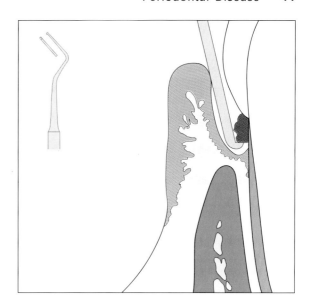

FIG. 5.9 Removing subgingival debris with a hoe.

depth excedes 4-6 mm), a flap is raised and 'open curettage' performed (see Fig. 5.14).

Root Planing

Root planing of any exposed or roughened root surfaces using the subgingival curette will produce a smooth root surface, free from debris and less likely to accumulate more. Numerous overlapping strokes are made, each time pulling the curette coronally out of the pocket, its cutting edge firmly engaged in the cementum of the root (Fig. 5.10).All the necrotic and diseased cementum is removed in this way. The outer edge of the curette engages any diseased pocket epithelium. As the curette is withdrawn, the diseased epithelium is removed. It may be necessary to apply light digital pressure to the gingiva, to hold the diseased gingiva against the curette.

To smooth the root surface numerous overlapping strokes in different directions are used, moving the curette diagonally (corono-rostrally and corono-caudally), horizontally (circumferentially) and vertically (coronally). When the root surface is smooth, the explorer is used to detect any remaining irregularities, which are removed with the curette.

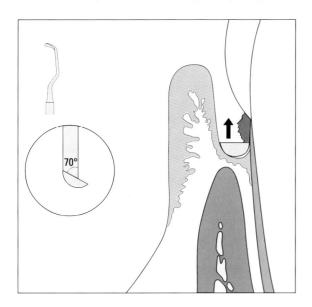

FIG. 5.8 Removing subgingival debris with a subgingival curette. Inset: Cross section of the curette's working tip, showing the angle of the cutting edges to the handle.

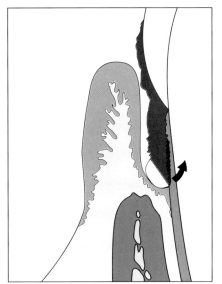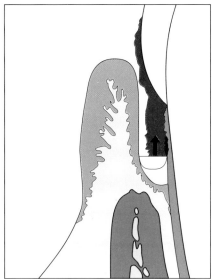

FIG. 5.10 Root planing. Left: The curette is inserted into the pocket with its curved edge against the epithelium. It is turned to engage the cutting edge in the necrotic cementum and debris. Right: The curette is withdrawn, removing the subgingival debris and necrotic cementum and scraping the pocket epithelium.

If the pathological pocket is more than 4 mm deep, 'open curettage' should be performed (see Fig. 5.14), raising a flap to allow proper access to the tooth structures to be cleaned. The flap may also need to be repositioned apically to eliminate the pocket. When a flap is raised, mechanical scalers may be used for root planing as the cooling water is able to reach the tip of the instrument.

Polishing

Polishing all the cleaned tooth surfaces is very important. Omitting this part of the scale and polish leaves the tooth surfaces roughened (Fig. 5.11), accelerating the rate of plaque adhesion and the continuing of periodontal disease. The prophy cup, the soft rubber polishing cup, is filled with fine grade fluoride polishing paste, or a plain flour pumice and water paste. Revolving at up to 1000 rpm, the cup is pressed lightly on to the tooth to flare out subgingivally (Fig. 5.12) and moved steadily over the tooth surface in a slurry of paste. All tooth surfaces are polished, paying particular attention to exposed root surfaces and the gingival margin.

Iatrogenic thermal damage will result if:

- insufficient prophy paste is used — refill the prophy cup when the slurry of prophy paste is diminishing, adding water if necessary
- over 1000 rpm is used — adjust the speed control to less than 1000 rpm
- excessive pressure is applied to flare out the prophy cup to polish subgingivally — buy softer prophy cups
- more than 15 seconds of continuous polishing is performed on one tooth — keep the prophy cup moving over the teeth; if a tooth is excessively stained, it may be necessary to return to it after it has cooled (10–20 seconds).

Sulcular Lavage

Sulcular lavage is the final stage of the non-surgical dental prophylaxis. Debris is flushed from the gingival crevice and pockets with dilute chlorhexidine or povidone–iodine from a 20–60 ml syringe. The stream of fluid is accurately directed subgingivally with a bluntened 21G needle or plastic pipette tip. It is not advisable to use pressurized water as this may embed infective particles in the inflamed tissues,

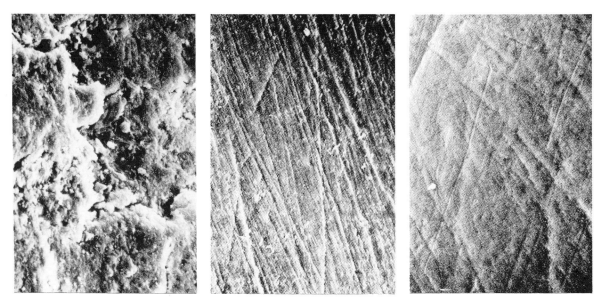

FIG. 5.11 Scanning electron micrographs of the enamel surface. Left: After ultrasonic scaling. Centre: After polishing with coarse pumice. Right: After the final polishing with fine pumice. Reproduced by kind permission of Dr U. B. Dietrich and the Veterinary Practice Publishing Company.

instead of flushing them away.

Post-operative antibiotics are rarely necessary after minor periodontal therapy.

Minor Periodontal Surgery

Basic Principles

When possible, a scale and polish is performed 2–3 weeks before the periodontal surgery is undertaken. A daily homecare regime is instigated, both to allow the tissues to heal in a clean environment and to test the client's ability and commitment to daily homecare. If the client is unable or unwilling to carry out homecare effectively, periodontal surgery will not provide a lasting result. Good homecare is essential for successful periodontal surgery.

Prior to periodontal surgery, a thorough scale and polish is performed and the mouth cleaned with chlorhexidine or povidone–iodine. Where infection exists, it is wise to instigate a course of antibiotics 5 days before surgery and to continue post operatively.

At least 2 mm of attached gingiva should remain post-operatively. Without attached gingiva, the alveolar mucosa and alveolar bone

recede rapidly, exposing the roots and leaving them unsupported. The tooth is then lost. When using thermocautery or electrosurgery to cut the gingiva, it is important to allow for the 1 mm or so of tissue that will slough post-operatively.

Gingiva is tough tissue. Sharp instruments are essential: scalpel blades must be renewed fre-

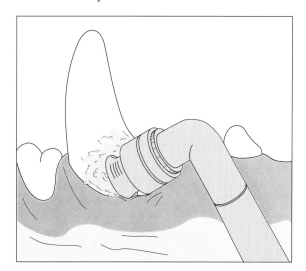

FIG. 5.12 Polishing the tooth surface, flaring the prophy cup subgingivally.

quently during each procedure; cutting needles with swaged on 4-0 absorbable suture material are preferable to round-bodied needles.

The normal anatomical features should be retained or recreated.

Pockets deeper than 4 mm may need attention. If there are no pathological changes, the pocket's depth should be noted and it should be checked every 6 months. If pathology has developed, a thorough scale and polish with root planing is essential, with minor periodontal surgery where appropriate, preceded and followed by rigorous homecare.

Post-operatively, soft foods and three times daily spraying or flushing of the surgical sites with 0.2% w/v chlorhexidine or an oral hygiene spray and application of chlorhexidine gel are advisable for 10–14 days. After this, daily toothbrushing with a firm but soft toothbrush and a flouride animal toothpaste will help to prevent periodontal disease from taking hold again.

Gingivoplasty

Gingivoplasty is the removal of diseased or excess gingival tissue to eliminate false or suprabony pockets, provided at least 2 mm of attached gingiva (coronal to the mucogingival line) remains post operatively. Its most common application is in the treatment of gingival hyperplasia or epulis.

The procedure is illustrated in Fig. 5.13.

1. Pocket depth is measured with a graduated periodontal probe (Fig. 5.13 a).
2. The probe is withdrawn from the pocket, held against the gingiva to show the depth of the pocket and its tip pressed into the gingiva at 90° to the tooth, to create a bleeding point (Fig. 5.13 a).
3. The process is repeated along the whole pocket.
4. A new size 15 scalpel blade or an electrosurgery, diathermy or thermocautery unit is used to make a bevelled incision, joining the bleeding points and recreating the scalloped edge of the normal gingival anatomy, taking care to leave at least 2 mm of attached gingiva *in situ* (Fig. 5.13 b).

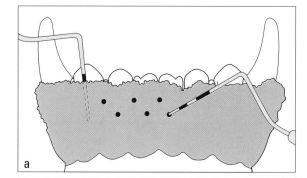
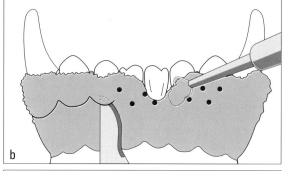
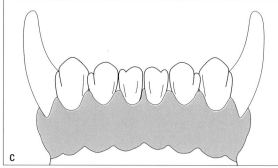

FIG. 5.13 Gingivoplasty of the lower incisor and canine gingival tissue. (a) Using the periodontal probe to measure and mark the pocket depth. (b) Making the bevelled incision. (c) The new, scalloped gingival margin.

Allow for the 1 mm slough if using heat to cut.
5. As attached gingiva is not elastic, it will not spring away once cut. Lift it off with forceps, a curette or a scaler.
6. Haemorrhage is controlled with gauze swabs and digital pressure.
7. The newly exposed tooth surface is then scaled and polished.

Gingivoplasty is contraindicated in areas with insufficient attached gingiva, or horizontal or vertical bone loss extending beyond the mucogingival line. Mucogingival surgery is the treatment of choice in these situations.

Mucogingival Surgery

Pathological pockets deeper than 4 mm with horizontal or vertical bone loss or less than 2 mm of attached gingiva are treated with a combination of procedures. Thorough subgingival cleaning (currettage and root planing) is essential. When the alveolar bone has been damaged by the disease process, it often needs to be remodelled to recreate the normal anatomy and eliminate any spicules or undermined bone, a procedure known as osteoplasty. These procedures are more easily performed properly when the gingiva has been reflected, improving both access and visibility. Where necessary, often when there is significant bone loss, the flap can then be repositioned apically, to avoid recreating the pocket. Procedures performed using a flap are termed open procedures, e.g. open curettage. It is important to remember that the base of a flap must not be any narrower than its free margin.

Open curettage with a simple flap

When the bone needs little remodelling (e.g. with minor horizontal bone loss) and the gingival margin does not need to be repositioned, this technique of minor flap surgery is employed. The procedure is illustrated in Fig. 5.14.

1. The epithelial attachment is cut using a size 15 scalpel blade, following the scalloped contours of the gingival margin (Fig. 5.14 a, b). Any diseased crevicular epithelium is also excised with this incision,

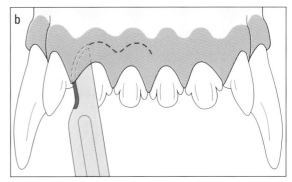

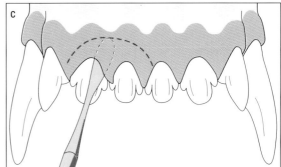

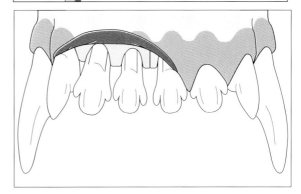

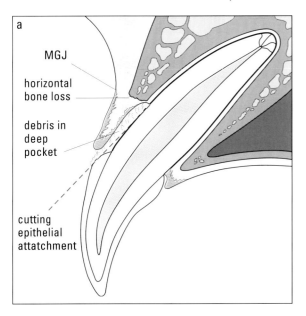

Fig. 5.14 Open curettage of the right upper central and intermediate incisors. (a) Cutting the epithelial attachment; longitudinal section. (b) The incision reaches the crestal alveolar bone. (c) The periosteal elevator is used to raise the attached gingiva. (d) The released gingiva is rolled back to expose the roots and crestal bone.

taking care to preserve the interdental papillae.

2. If a large subgingival area is to be exposed, a vertical releasing incision is made at each end of the initial, horizontal incision. These should not extend beyond the mucogingival line, because only the interdental papillae and part of the attached gingiva are reflected, and the flap is to be replaced in its original position.

3. A small, sharp periosteal elevator is used to separate the periosteum and attached gingiva from the coronal 1–2 mm of crestal alveolar bone (Fig. 5.14 c).

4. The released gingiva is then rolled back, exposing the roots and crestal alveolar bone (Fig. 5.14 d).

5. Fine, sharp subgingival curettes are used to remove remnants of pocket epithelium, granulation tissue, necrotic cementum and debris from the surface of the tooth. Thorough, systematic root planing is performed with repeated irrigation; this is the most important part of the procedure.

6. Any bony defects are removed with a low-speed, round-headed bur and constant irrigation with a copious flow of sterile saline. This is minor osteoplasty.

7. The cleaned and root-planed tooth surfaces are carefully polished.

8. The whole area is flushed with dilute chlorhexidine or povidone–iodine, then sterile saline, to remove any debris.

9. The flap is lain back in its original position. This may mean that the attached gingiva is placed partly over bone and partly over tooth root, potentially recreating a pocket. The attached gingiva will reattach itself to the underlying bone, provided the area is completely clean. A long junctional epithelial attachment usually forms to join the coronal attached gingiva to the underlying tooth root. This is a relatively weak attachment. Thorough homecare is critical for success and usually eliminates the recreation of pockets.

10. The flap is adapted to the underlying bone and the necks of the teeth. Digital pressure is applied to the area for one minute, to eliminate dead space and increase the chances of gingival reattachment. It is not usually necessary to suture the flap in place if releasing incisions were not made. However, if releasing incisions were made, the interdental papillae, which were carefully preserved during the scalloping of the initial incision, are used to close the flap over the interdental areas without tension, using single interrupted sutures of absorbable suture material swaged on to a cutting needle. The releasing incisions are closed in a similar fashion.

Open curettage with an apically repositioned flap

When there are pockets deeper than 6 mm with marked alveolar bone loss, the chances of complete gingival reattachment, in its original position post-operatively, are minimal. If the attached gingiva is moved apically so that some of it lies over healthy bone, reattachment is more successful, reducing the risk of pocket recreation. The procedure is illustrated in Fig. 5.15.

1. The epithelial attachment is cut using a size 15 scalpel blade, following the scalloped contours of the gingival margin (Fig. 5.15 a). Any diseased crevicular epithelium is also excised with this incision, taking care to preserve the interdental papillae.

2. As the flap is to be repositioned apically, and a large subgingival area is to be exposed, a vertical releasing incision is made at each end of the initial, horizontal incision. These extend into the alveolar mucosa to allow the flap to be repositioned apically (Fig. 5.15 b).

3. A small, sharp periosteal elevator is used to separate the periosteum and attached gingiva from the underlying alveolar bone, extending beyond the mucogingival line (Fig. 5.15 c). It is sometimes easier to raise the flap by inserting the periosteal elevator under the gingiva at the releasing incision and working it between the periosteum and

the alveolar bone, from the releasing incision along the flap and coronally. This full-thickness gingival flap (including periosteum) is then reflected. A lingual flap is raised in the same way if there is pathology lingually.

4. Fine, sharp subgingival curettes are used to remove remnants of pocket epithelium, granulation tissue, necrotic cementum and debris from the surface of the tooth. Thorough, systematic root planing is performed with repeated irrigation; this is the most important part of the procedure.

5. Where there are bony defects or vertical bony pockets, these defects and partially eroded spicules of bone are removed with a low-speed, round-headed bur and constant irrigation with a copious flow of

sterile saline. This is osteoplasty. Any bulbous bony margins are also eliminated, particularly on the facial surface between teeth, by narrowing the buccal and lingual cortical plates. This facilitates the

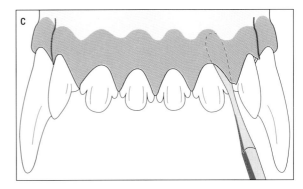

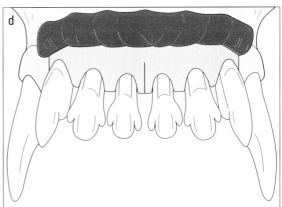

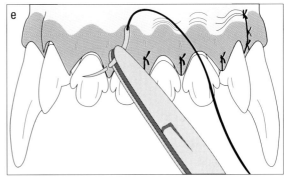

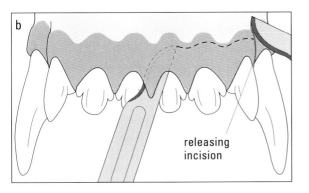

Fig. 5.15 Apically repositioned flap involving the gingiva of the upper incisors. (a) Cutting the epithelial attachment; longitudinal section. (b) The horizontal incision reaches the crestal alveolar bone; the releasing incision extends beyond the MGJ. (c) The periosteal elevator is used to raise the attached gingiva. (d) The released gingiva is rolled back to expose the roots and alveolar bone. (e) The flap is repositioned and sutured.

subsequent replacement of the flap and the regeneration of the physiological morphology of the gingival margin.

6. The cleaned and root-planed tooth surfaces are carefully polished.
7. The whole area is flushed with dilute chlorhexidine or povidone–iodine, then sterile saline, to remove any debris.
8. The flap is positioned as required (Fig. 5.15 e). Generally, the free gingival margin is placed 2 mm coronal to the margin of the alveolar bone, completely covering the alveolar bone. The attached gingiva will then reattach itself to the underlying bone. If there has been marked bone loss, or if the alveolar bone margin has been remodelled and moved apically by osteoplasty, as with the vertical bone loss associated with infrabony pockets, the re-positioning of the flap apically should prevent the recreation of pockets. The alveolar mucosa will wrinkle to accommodate the excess tissue.

It is essential that the gingival margin of the flap is coronal to the mucogingival line of the adjacent gingiva, to ensure that attached gingiva heals to attached gingiva, and that there is no gap in the attached gingiva. This may mean that the attached gingiva is placed partly over bone and partly over tooth root, potentially recreating a pocket. The apical attached gingiva should reattach to the underlying alveolar bone. Usually, a long junctional epithelial attachment forms between the remaining attached gingiva and the tooth root throughout the depth of this potential pocket. This is a relatively weak attachment, so thorough homecare is critical for its success. The formation of these reattachments is dependent on the absolute cleanliness of the surfaces concerned, so thorough root planing, curettage and removal of diseased pocket epithelium are essential.

9. The labial and palatal flaps are adapted to the underlying bone and the necks of the teeth. The interdental papillae, which were

carefully preserved during the scalloping of the initial incision, are used to close the flaps over the interdental areas without tension, using single interrupted sutures of absorbable suture material swaged onto a cutting needle. The releasing incisions are closed in a similar fashion. Digital pressure is applied to the area for one minute to eliminate dead space and improve the chances of reattachment.

Splinting

Avulsed teeth and incisors which have suffered sufficient periodontal disease and bone loss to render them unstable, may be saved by splinting them together, using the nearest firm teeth (i.e. canines or lateral incisors) as end-posts. Thin, orthodontic or orthopaedic wire or colourless, monofilament nylon and transparent or enamel-coloured, non-exothermic, dental acrylic are used. Thorough homecare is essential; any debris allowed to accumulate will interfere with the healing process, preventing regeneration and reattachment of the periodontal tissues.

The procedure is preceded by a thorough scale and polish, with root planing and open curettage where necessary, with devoted homecare and antibiotics as required. After approximately 2 weeks, when the disease processes are under control and the client has shown the ability to clean the teeth, the splint may be applied.

Procedure

1. The teeth to be splinted are scaled and polished.
2. The subgingival area is thoroughly cleaned again, taking care not to destroy healthy, healing tissue.
3. The area to be splinted is measured and an appropriate length of fine ligature wire cut.
4. The ligature wire is woven in a figure-of-eight fashion along the incisors, using the lateral incisors as anchors, if they are firm enough, or the canines if all the incisors are loose.

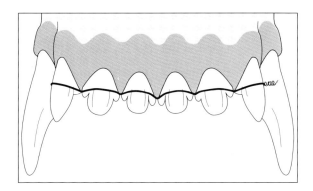

FIG. 5.16 Figure-of-eight wire in place for splinting incisors.

5. The figure-of-eight wire is tightened with a haemostat at the distal end of one of the anchor teeth (Fig. 5.16).

6. The end is cut and the pigtail tucked in behind the tooth to prevent soft tissue trauma.

7. The teeth are acid etched, on the labial and lingual surfaces of all the teeth to be splinted. The etchant is rinsed off, taking care to protect the soft tissues, following the manufacturer's instructions.

8. The liquid acrylic monomer and the powder polymer are placed in separate dappen dishes.

9. A brush is soaked in the liquid, dabbed into the powder and applied to the etched tooth surfaces, including the wire. A thin but complete layer is applied. It is essential to prevent the acrylic from flowing into the gingival crevice or on to exposed root surfaces as this will further damage the periodontium and reduce the chances of regeneration and reattachment of the periodontal tissues. When using monofilament nylon, this is applied to the teeth in the same 'figure of eight' format immediately after the first layer of acrylic has been applied, and held in place whilst the acrylic sets. Whilst the surgeon is holding the nylon still, an assistant can apply further layers of acrylic.

10. Additional layers of acrylic are applied, using the soak-and-dab technique already described, to form a band 2–4 mm high and 2–3 mm thick around the teeth.

11. The splint is shaped while the acrylic is still soft, to follow the anatomical configuration of the teeth. It is essential that the splint does not interfere with occlusion and that there is sufficient space between the splint and the soft tissues to allow for proper oral hygiene.

12. The splint is shaped, smoothed and polished, using a slow handpiece and acrylic burs if available ensuring that there is nowhere for debris to accumulate.

13. After 2-4 months, some periodontal repair will have occurred. The splint may then be replaced by a lighter version. If the teeth are left unsplinted, they will tend to migrate out of proper alignment, due to a lack of bony support. An excellent standard of oral hygiene is essential.

Emily splint

An Emily splint is an adaptation of this technique, where threaded orthodontic wire or several TMS pins are attached to the lingual surfaces of the teeth using composite or acrylic. Being only on the lingual surfaces of the teeth, this splint is less likely to interfere with the gingiva and is aesthetically more acceptable than the figure-of-eight splint.

Emily splint procedure

1. A shallow groove is drilled along the lingual surfaces of all the teeth to be splinted using the edge of a $33\frac{1}{2}$ inverted cone bur. The groove runs horizontally approximately at the level of the cingulae of the incisors (Fig. 5.17), which is the area of greatest contact between the teeth and is far enough away from the gingiva to avoid gingival damage.

2. If threaded orthodontic wire is to be used, it is bent to follow the shape of the lingual surfaces of the incisors exactly, so that it will lie in the groove. If it is not bent accurately, the teeth will be moved towards the wire. As this wire is hard to find, a practical alternative is to use the working

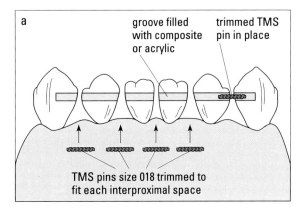

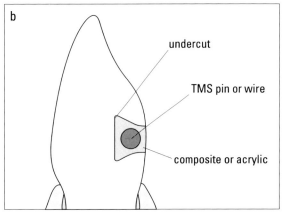

Fig. 5.17 The Emily splint. (a) Lingual view. Trimmed TMS pins being placed in the groove filled with composite or acrylic. (b) Side view. Cross-section of TMS pin or wire in place in the groove on the lingual surface of an incisor

end of an old Hedstrom file, with the handle end removed. TMS pins are very short and do not need to be bent, but they may need to be trimmed to fit the interproximal space (Fig. 5.17). The working end of an old Hedstrom file can be cut into short sections which can be used as TMS pins. The ridges on the threaded wire, the Hedstrom file and the TMS pins help to hold the splint together, increasing the stability of the splint.

3.   The groove and the lingual tooth surface to 1 mm each side of the groove are acid etched and rinsed, according to the manufacturer's instructions.
4.   Unfilled resin, adhesive or acrylic is painted on to the etched surface and cured or air dried, following the manufacturer's instructions.
5.   Composite or acrylic is placed in the groove.
6.   The bent wire is pressed into the composite or acrylic in the groove. This forces composite or acrylic into the undercuts in the teeth. If TMS pins are used, a pin is pressed into the composite or acrylic in the groove at the edges of two neighbouring teeth, so that it lies across the gap between the teeth, thus holding them together (Fig. 5.17). Further pins are placed between the remaining teeth to be splinted.
7.   The composite or acrylic is cured. Remember that if light-cured composite is used, the light will not be able to penetrate the wire or pins to cure the composite below. Several light-cured composites will cure chemically if they are not cured properly by the light, so it is important to use a composite with a chemical curing facility, or a chemically cured composite.
8.   Further composite or acrylic is applied and cured, to create a thin, smooth band which completely covers the wire or pins and attaches to the tooth on each side of the wire or pins. It should not contact the gingiva anywhere, nor should it interfere with the occlusion.
9.   If necessary, the splint is shaped, using a finishing bur, and polished.
10. The composite is acid etched, rinsed, dried and coated with a thin layer of unfilled resin which is then cured. This gives the splint a very smooth surface which will be less likely to attract plaque and debris.
11. Daily toothbrushing and flushing with an oral hygiene solution (e.g. a palatable chlorhexidine gluconate solution) will help to maintain an excellent standard of oral hygiene, which is essential.

Odontoplasty

Odontoplasty is strictly the removal of tooth structure; however, the term is sometimes applied to the removal of excess filling material or reshaping ill-fitting cast crowns. When gingival and alveolar bony recession have exposed part of the tooth root, plaque and debris tend to accumulate between the enamel bulge and the gingival margin. In order to prevent further progression of the periodontal disease, this debris must be prevented from accumulating.

The easiest and least traumatic method of removing this debris is to brush the teeth daily, paying particular attention to affected teeth. Constant removal of the debris will prevent it from accumulating. It has been suggested that removing the enamel bulge, followed by daily toothbrushing, is a more permanent cure. Once removed, however, there is nothing to protect the gingival margin. Anything chewed is driven into the gingival crevice, physically forcing further gingival recession and introducing debris subgingivally (Fig. 5.18). The dentine exposed by this procedure is sensitive and should be treated with fluoride in an attempt to reduce this sensitivity. Exposure of the dentine may lead to tooth mortality.

If owners are able to brush their pets' teeth, it is better to leave the enamel bulge in place so it can continue to protect the gingivae. If toothbrushing is not possible, it is inevitable that affected teeth will be lost. Without the

protection of the enamel bulge, it is likely that the gingivae will recede and the teeth will be lost more quickly than if the enamel bulge were able to continue its function.

Some feel that the lips and cheeks play an important role in the constant removal of debris from the outer surfaces of the teeth. The removal of the enamel bulge coronal to an area of gingival recession is thought to allow the lips and cheeks to come into contact with the whole tooth surface, thus constantly wiping it clean. In normal teeth, this method of 'self-cleaning' is not successful, so in an already compromised tooth, it is unlikely to be more sucessful.

Odontoplasty may be used to remove dental anomalies, such as irregular enamel projections, if they are creating a problem, a rare occurrence. Using coarse diamond or plain-cut tapered fissure burs in a high-speed handpiece, with water coolant, the overhanging buccal enamel projections or irregularities are removed, carefully creating a normal enamel bulge. Fine diamond burs are then used to smooth the surface. A fine abrasive rubber wheel is used for final polishing, in a low-speed handpiece with light pressure to reduce the risks of overheating the tooth and causing pulpal necrosis. Fluoride varnish is then applied over the tooth.

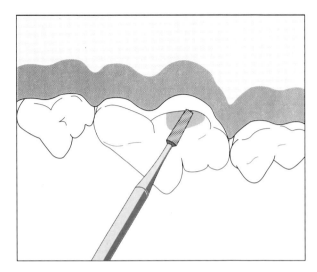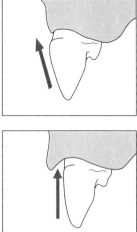

FIG. 5.18 Odontoplasty of the upper fourth premolar. Left: Removal of the enamel bulge with a plain cut tapered fissure bur. Top right: Enamel bulge deflecting food from the receded gingiva. Bottom right: Without the enamel bulge, food is driven on to the gingiva, exacerbating the gingival recession.

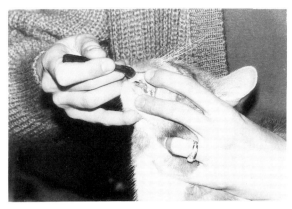

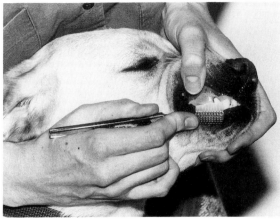

Fig. 5.19 Toothbrushing. Top: Brushing a cat's teeth with a soft cat toothbrush. Bottom: Brushing a dog's teeth.

Homecare

Animal teeth need to be kept clean just like our own. On a natural diet, chewing through thick skins and tough meat removes most of the plaque. However, this is not a significant part of our pets' diets. In order to prevent the otherwise inevitable progress of periodontal disease, pet owners must intervene. Feeding large pieces of raw vegetable (e.g. cauliflower, broccoli. cabbage or swede; gravy enhances the taste) or lightly cooked tough, fibrous meat (e.g. bovine trachea, diaphragm or heart) at least twice a week helps to wipe off the plaque, but there is really no substitute for daily toothbrushing with an animal toothpaste.

The physical removal of plaque with a soft but firm toothbrush is the most effective means of preventing periodontal disease (Fig. 5.19).

To complement this, some toothpastes contain fluoride and some of the enzymes and substrates of saliva, which augment its natural antibacterial properties. Used daily, from 3 months of age, the combination of effective toothbrushing, which massages the gums as well as cleaning the teeth, the fluoride and the antibacterial properties of some animal toothpastes should prevent most periodontal disease. Brushing also increases owners' awareness of their pets' mouths. They are more likely to notice oral lesions, such as fractured teeth, dental erosions, carious decay, malocclusions and soft tissue lesions, early enough for straightforward treatment to be instigated, if they are examining their pets' mouths daily.

After periodontal surgery or when brushing is not tolerated, spraying with an oral hygiene spray or applying 0.2% w/v chlorhexidine on a cotton bud will help to maintain oral hygiene.

Chronic Feline Stomatitis Gingivitis Complex

Some practical tips on treating this frustrating condition will be outlined here.

- Perform a thorough dental scale and polish, paying particular attention to the subgingival area. Apply fluoride foam or varnish to the cleaned teeth, followed by homecare to maintain oral hygiene.
- Treat any feline subgingival resorptive lesions as appropriate.
- Test for FIV, FCV and FeLV as these are implicated in the aetiology of this condition. Routine haematology and blood biochemistry tests are usually indicated.
- Supply antibiotics to eliminate both aerobic and anaerobic bacteria; a 3-week course is usually necessary (e.g. clindamycin).
- Apply a palatable 0.12% chlorhexidine gluconate gel to the gums 2–3 times daily. This is a very effective way of medicating the gingivae.
- Salicylic acid (aspirin) is usually effective in reducing the inflammation. A low dose given systemically is tolerated by cats ($\frac{1}{4}$ x 300 mg tablet every second day in food), but an

aspirin gel applied to the gingivae is much more effective. The dose rate is 25 mg/kg/day for 4 weeks, reducing to once every 2–3 days for maintenance, increasing again for short periods as necessary. There is no such gel on the market at present, but a pharmacist can make it up for you.

- Hyperplastic gingiva is removed to eliminate the false pockets (Fig. 5.13), taking great care to leave at least 2 mm of attached gingiva.
- Spray, bathe or gently brush the gingivae with 0.2% w/v chlorhexidine or an oral hygiene spray, which can be sprayed directly on to the gums, painted on with a cotton bud or brushed on with an extremely soft cat toothbrush. If brushing is possible, a fluoride enzymatic animal toothpaste is preferable to the spray.
- Supply vitamin and mineral supplements, particularly vitamin C and zinc.
- Bathe gingivae with *Lactobacillus* spp.; adding this to the food is the simplest method, using live natural yoghurt or *Lactobacillus* powder.
- Administer corticosteroids, preferably by long-acting depot injections, depending on the cat's viral status.
- Minor cryosurgery of the affected gingivae may help, but as it often results in the destruction of the attached gingiva by over-freezing, this technique is not recommended.
- If all else fails, extract the molars, premolars and incisors, ensuring absolutely no root fragments remain. If this fails, take radiographs to check for root fragments and remove them. As a last resort, if the condition still fails to respond, extract the canines. It has been said that if all the teeth are extracted entirely, the condition will be cured. This is still a subject of great debate. Toothless animals are less able to groom themselves, so devoted nursing is essential. Soft food is usually managed, but the face needs regular washing.

Feline oral disease will be covered in detail in the *Handbook of Advanced Small Animal Dentistry*, Penman, Emily and Gorrel (1994), Pergamon Press, in preparation.

6
Restorative Dentistry

The aim of restorative dental work in the human field is to replace lost tooth structure with an aesthetically pleasing, strong material, restoring the original anatomical features of the tooth. In animal dentistry, the aims are similar but modified. It is rarely practical to rebuild a tooth to its original size, as the forces of mastication would destroy most of the superfluous restorative material. Restorative materials are not as strong as the original tooth components. Veterinary dental restorative work is generally more concerned with function than aesthetics, so the use of materials to build up tooth structure beyond that remaining is usually avoided. The dental restorations of most use in veterinary dentistry are of teeth damaged by caries, resorptive lesions, erosions, enamel defects, and after the endodontic treatment of fractured teeth. These and the most commonly used materials and techniques of relevance to veterinary dentistry will be described in this chapter. Restorative dentistry is an enormous and rapidly evolving subject. New materials are being developed at such a rate that it is essential to follow the manufacturer's instructions.

Materials

The success of restorative dentistry depends upon the correct choice, understanding and use of materials. The manufacturers supply detailed instructions for the use of each material; these should be followed meticulously. New products are being developed at a prodigious rate, with various new properties, expanding the already enormous range of materials available. The three types of material used are metal alloys (amalgam), resin-based restoratives (composites) and glass-ionomer cements.

Amalgam

Amalgam is a silver–tin–copper alloy which combines with mercury to form the solid amalgam alloy. It has been used to fill cavities in human teeth for many years. It is usually held in place mechanically. An undercut is drilled in the tooth so that the bottom of the cavity is wider than the top. The cavity is lined to prevent microleakage of the toxic amalgam components and to provide thermal insulation. Once set, the amalgam should not fall out. Amalgam is the hardest dental restorative material, with the greatest resistance to wear, but when it is not attached to the tooth structure, it cannot impart any strength to the tooth. In fact, the removal of tooth structure when creating the retentive undercut weakens the tooth. Specialized equipment is also required to mix and handle amalgam. Where aesthetics are important, the silver colour of amalgam is undesirable. For these and other reasons, amalgam has largely been superceded by composites and glass-ionomers. The recent development of amalgam bonding agents which stick amalgam to the tooth structure makes amalgam a more useful restorative material.

Composite

Composite is a resin combined with inorganic filler particles to form a filled resin. The sizes of the particles vary from 0.04 to 5.0 μm. To gain the advantages of both extremes of size, hybrid composites with various combinations of particle sizes are used. These are strong composites with a fine surface finish and good resistance to wear.

Composite is cured either chemically or with

light. Chemically cured base and catalyst composite pastes are mixed together on a pad to initiate a chemical setting reaction which is completed at a predetermined rate. Light-cured composite is supplied as a paste in a light-proof syringe; the paste is cured by exposing it to light of 470 nm wavelength for 10–60 seconds. The setting reaction is faster and more easily controlled than for the chemically cured pastes. Eugenol prevents composite from setting, so it is important to remember never to use eugenol immediately under composite.

Various bonding agents are available for bonding composite to tooth structure. This reduces the need for undercuts, but it is still recommended that minimal undercuts are made to provide some mechanical retention to complement the bonding action. There are numerous different bonding agents, each with its own special technique, so it is essential to follow the manufacturer's instructions precisely. A bonding agent is applied to the dentine. The enamel is etched with phosphoric acid to open the hydroxyapatite lattice, and thoroughly rinsed. Unfilled resin is brushed on to the etched enamel and the dentine, then cured. The unfilled resin runs into and fills the open lattice of the etched enamel. It also bonds with the composite (filled resin) which is placed on top and cured. The composite is thus firmly bonded to the tooth structure, enabling the composite to impart some strength to the tooth.

Composites are available in various tooth-coloured shades, but even the lightest shade is often slightly darker than animal enamel. They are also supplied in 'dentine' or 'enamel'; the 'dentine' composite is more opaque than the translucent 'enamel' composite.

Glass-Ionomer Cements

Glass-ionomer cements consist of a polyalkenoic acid and ion-leachable fluoride aluminosilicate glass particles. They set hard when mixed with water or a solution of tartaric acid. As the initial setting reaction requires a tiny amount of water at the tooth/cement interface, the prepared tooth surface is not dried completely but left slightly dewy. Since the reaction is susceptible to excess water, which would wash out essential cement-forming ions, a varnish is applied immediately after placing the cement to protect the surface from exposure to saliva (and also from dehydration) during setting.

Glass-ionomers bond directly to both enamel and dentine, reducing the need for undercuts or etching and imparting some strength to the tooth structure. They also leach fluoride ions into the surrounding tooth structure; these ions are anticariogenic (inhibit the formation of caries) and strengthen enamel and dentine.

Unfortunately, these cements are weak in compression and should not be used on occlusal surfaces. They are commonly used in the repair of feline subgingival resorptive lesions, which rarely involve occlusal surfaces, and in the repair of carious lesions, in direct contact with the affected tooth surface and overlain with composite or amalgam to provide compressive strength on occlusal surfaces. To improve the strength and resistance to abrasion of the glass-ionomer cements, cermet–ionomer cements were developed by sintering metal (usually silver) to the glass particles. These materials are still not strong enough to resist the forces of occlusion, but research is continuing.

There are three types of glass-ionomer cement:

- Type I: luting cements, used for sticking on crowns and veneers
- Type II: restorative materials:
  (i) aesthetic (tooth-coloured)
  (ii) reinforced (including silver–cermet-ionomer cements)
- Type III: fast-setting lining materials and fissure sealants.

The precise type chosen depends on the use for which it is required. Types II and III are often used as liners and dentine adhesives under composite, as glass-ionomers can be etched, and as liners under amalgam.

Glass-ionomers are available as a powder and a liquid which are mixed together, or in a precapsulated form (applicaps) which is mixed

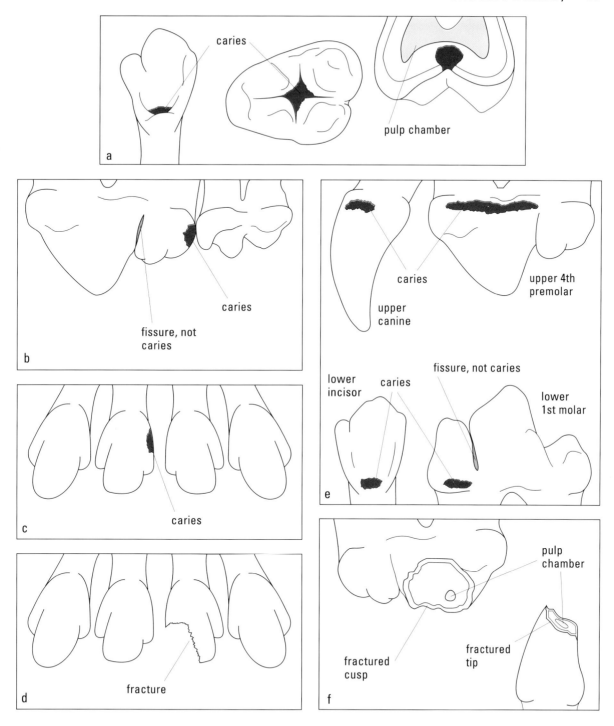

FIG. 6.1 Classification of cavities. (a) Class I: left: lower incisor, lingual view; rarely involved; centre: upper first molar, occlusal view; commonly affected; right: section through an upper first molar, showing the extent of the decay often found. (b) Class II: caries between the upper fourth premolar and the first molar; rarely seen in animals. (c) Class III: caries between central incisors; rare in animals. (d) Class IV: fracture of an incisor involving part of the incisal edge; common in animals. (e) Class V: labial aspects of teeth commonly affected. (f) Class VI: the most common cavity in animals; left: fractured upper fourth premolar with the loss of the rostral cusp as a 'slab fracture'; right: fractured lower canine.

in a glass-ionomer activator (a machine similar to an amalgamator). Light cured glass-ionomers are also available.

Cavities

The boundaries and extents of cavities can be classified according to their type and position, after a human classification system (Fig. 6.1).

Class I   Cavities beginning in structural defects in the teeth (pits and fissures). This is a common site of decay, particularly for caries in the dog.

Class II Cavities in the proximal surfaces of (i.e. between) the molars and premolars usually at contact points. This type of cavity is rarely seen in dogs and cats.

Class III Cavities in the proximal surfaces of (i.e. between) the incisors and canines which do not involve the removal and restoration of the incisal angle. These lesions are rarely seen in the dog and cat.

Class IV Cavities in the proximal surfaces of the incisors and canines which require the removal and restoration of the incisal angle. These are common in fractures of the front teeth in the dog and cat.

Class V   Cavities in the gingival third of the labial or lingual surfaces of the teeth, not involving pits or fissures. These are common sites of lesions in the dog and cat and are associated with habitually unclean areas of the teeth.

Class VI Cavities in the incisal edge of the anterior teeth or the cusp tips in the posterior teeth. This is the commonest cavity in the dog and cat, and often involves the fracture of a cusp tip, particularly of the canines and upper fourth premolars.

Caries

Dental decay or caries can occur on any tooth surface. It usually begins with the

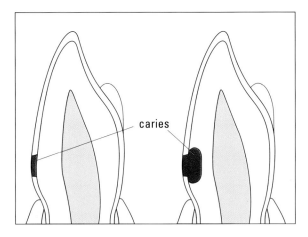

Fig. 6.2 The progression of dental decay: longitudinal sections of a lower first molar. Left: An early lesion involving only the enamel. Right: The progression of decay through the enamel and into the dentine, not exposing the pulp.

demineralization of the enamel, visible as a discoloration. The enamel is the only protection the tooth has from decay; once its integrity has been broken and the dentine exposed, the carious breakdown of the dentine ensues (Fig. 6.2). This is an organic decay and proceeds much faster than the inorganic demineralization of the enamel. Exposed root structure has no enamel covering and is very susceptible to decay.

Caries is grossly underdiagnosed in dogs, largely because it is difficult to detect in conscious animals. It is most commonly found on the grinding surfaces of the molars, particularly in the larger breeds. An estimated 40% of British dogs have caries.

Clinically, early caries is visible as a small dark brown or black spot in the enamel. A sharp instrument (e.g. Shepherd's hook explorer or 23 gauge needle) will stick in the lesion. A small enamel defect usually covers a large cavern of decayed dentine. As dentine decays so rapidly, restoration should be performed immediately. Radiography is used to determine the extent of the lesion and hence the most appropriate treatment. If the pulp is involved, endodontic treatment is indicated, but if too much tooth structure has been lost, extraction may be necessary.

Caries in animals can be a very painful

process, as it is in humans, although the clinical signs of dental pain in animals are often so subtle, insidious in onset and not exclusively oral, that they are missed. Common signs include:

- dysphagia, particularly with hard food; may chew on one side
- excessive salivation
- pawing at the mouth: rubbing the mouth and face along the ground
- 'premature ageing'
- change in temperament; may become aggressive and resent patting on the head; may become dull and lethargic, hiding away, unwilling to play.

It is often only with hindsight, after the treatment of dental lesions and the animal's return to normality, that the degree of dental pain the animal had been suffering can be appreciated. The animals rely on us to look for such lesions constantly, without waiting for symptoms.

Feline Subgingival Resorptive Lesions

Feline subgingival resorptive lesions or 'neck lesions' are erosions in the tooth at the cemento-enamel junction. They are not carious. Cellular digestion of the dental tissues by multinucleated giant cells analogous to odontoclasts and osteoclasts creates neck lesions, which are lined by these cells. Inflamed, hyperplastic gingiva containing multi-nucleated giant cells fills the lesion.

An estimated 57% of British cats are affected, with the number of teeth involved varying from 1 to 11. The premolars and molars are most commonly affected, although lesions are seen in the canines and incisors. The lesions are most common in young adult domestic cats and seem to be related to periodontal disease and soft foods.

Neck lesions are extremely painful, although there may be few clinical signs, as desribed in the previous section under 'Caries'. A diagnosis is reached after:

- visual inspection; the erosion itself may be visible, but more often, the associated

hyperplastic gingiva can be seen
- tactile exploration with a Shepherd's hook explorer; the instrument does not stick as it does in soft carious tooth substance, but grates on the hard rough edges and surface of the lesion
- radiography; the full extent of the lesion and hence an accurate diagnosis can only be achieved radiographically.

Feline subgingival resorptive lesions can be classified into five categories, each of which has a different approach to treatment. Proper treatment depends on the accurate classification of these lesions. Good radiographs are essential for the definitive diagnosis of neck lesions.

The five categories of feline subgingival resorptive lesions are:

Class I   extends to less than 0.5 mm depth
Class II   deeper than 0.5 mm but does not invade the pulp chamber
Class III   deep erosion invading the pulp chamber
Class IV   erosion creates a physical separation between the crown and the root, the floating crown
Class V   complete loss of crown with root retention and subsequent gingival overgrowth.

The treatment depends on the classification of the lesion.

Class I lesions are too small to restore, so treatment is aimed at preventing further odontoclastic activity. A meticulous scale and polish is performed, including thorough subgingival curettage, root planing, polishing and sulcular lavage. Any hyperplastic gingiva in the lesion (which houses many differentiating multi-nucleated giant cells) should be removed with a scalpel. The application of a fluoride foam or varnish helps to desensitize the dentine and to harden the enamel, which is thought to slow the progress of the lesion. A record is kept of the oral pathology and its treatment on a dental recording chart (see Fig.1.9).

Homecare is vital; without it, the progress of the lesion will not be halted. The owner is shown how to brush the teeth daily with an animal toothpaste containing fluoride and a cat toothbrush. The diet is changed to dry food. Also, feeding the cat 4 oz of lightly boiled fibrous meat (e.g. heart) twice daily may be beneficial. A detailed re-examination after 3–6 months is recommended.

Class II lesions can be restored. It is debatable whether removing the hyperplastic gingiva and filling the defect halts the progression of the lesion. As glass-ionomers leach fluoride, they are probably the material of choice. A technique for the restoration of Class II lesions is described in detail later in this chapter.

Class III lesions involve the pulp and so necessitate endodontic treatment prior to restoration. In practice, this means that only the canine teeth are treated. Premolars and molars with Class III lesions should be extracted very carefully, as teeth with such deep erosions fracture very easily.

Class IV lesions cannot be restored. Affected teeth are extracted, ensuring that all the roots are removed entirely.

Class V lesions are detected radiographically. The retained roots are extracted if they are causing a problem.

Cavity Preparation

The general principles of cavity preparation are the same for all types of cavity, but there is no specific design of cavity preparation to suit all cavities. Each cavity preparation should be designed individually to repair the particular defect. The main aims are to maintain the integrity of the pulp and to preserve healthy tooth substance. The important points to remember are:

• the enamel rods are arranged at right angles to the tooth surface; any unsupported enamel at the surface of a restoration (i.e. edges or portions of unsupported or undermined enamel rods) will break off, leaving a gap in the restoration for debris to accumulate, resulting in the failure of the restoration
• the undercut is made in the dentine, to retain the restorative material
• the pulp must be protected from irritation

caused by the restorative material or external stimuli, either by an adequate thickness of dentine (at least 2 mm) or by an insulating base and cavity liner (e.g. glass-ionomer on top of calcium hydroxide cement)
• the decayed area is removed without weakening the tooth structure and without penetrating the pulp, preserving as much of the inherently strong tooth structure as possible, as filling material is not as strong as healthy tooth substance
• the cavity preparation is designed to facilitate filling and finishing, minimizing the weaknesses of the restorative material.

Procedure

The procedures for preparing cavities are illustrated in Fig. 6.3.

1. The teeth are cleaned and polished with a non-fluoride pumice, and the lesion explored with an explorer.
2. A radiograph is taken to determine the extent of the lesion and the existence of complicating factors (e.g. apical pathology); if there is pulpal involvement, endodontic therapy or extraction is indicated.
3. The carious dentine and debris are removed with a dental spoon excavator, being careful to avoid penetrating the pulp of deeper lesions.
4. A pear-shaped or round bur is used to remove any remaining carious dentine, taking great care to avoid pulpal involvement.
5. A small undercut is made in the dentine with a small pear-shaped or round bur. The inverted cone bur is used less often than previously, as it creates too sharp an angle along the deep margin of the cavity. This prevents the filling materials being pressed right in, automatically resulting in a void around the deep margin of the cavity. A curved undercut is easily filled completely.
6. Any unsupported enamel is removed, by running a dental spoon excavator, a clean supragingival scaler or a long, pear-shaped or straight fissure bur around the enamel margin of the cavity preparation. Where

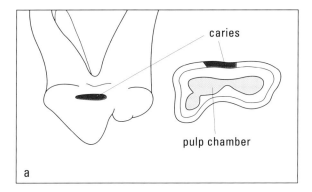
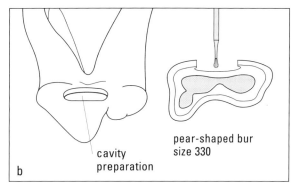
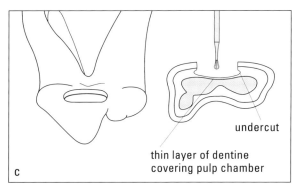
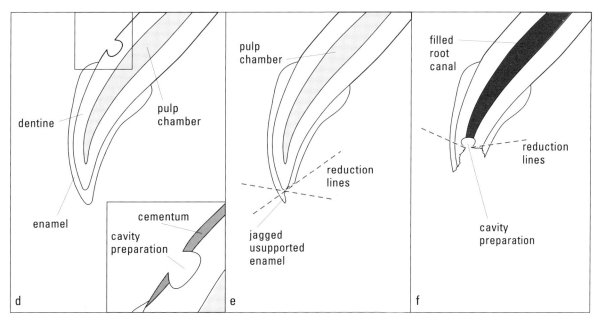

FIG. 6.3 Cavity preparations; note the vertical enamel margins and that the undercut is in the dentine. (a) Early Class V carious cavity of an upper fourth premolar. (b) Cavity preparation, showing the undercut in the dentine. (c) Deep Class V cavity preparation of an upper fourth premolar, not exposing the pulp. (d) Root cavity (e.g. feline subgingival resorptive lesion); longitudinal section. (e) Minor Class VI cavity not exposing the pulp; longitudinal section. (f) Class VI cavity after root canal therapy to treat the exposed pulp; longitudinal section.

the tooth has been fractured, the jagged edges are removed, recreating a tooth shape where possible (following the reduction lines, Figs 6.3e and f). Sharp edges are smoothed, using a long, pear-shaped bur or a sanding disc. There may be no need for further restoration (e.g. the fracture of the canine tip, not involving the pulp in Fig. 6.3d).

7. If the cavity preparation is to be filled (i.e. all cavities except Fig. 6.3d), it is thoroughly flushed clean with pressurized water, then dried.

Filling the Prepared Cavity

Dental materials are being developed at a very fast rate, hence the exact details of the techniques for each material are changing. It is essential that the manufacturer's instructions are followed precisely as there are many variations of the basic procedures detailed below.

Using Composite

A superficial cavity

The procedure is illustrated in Fig. 6.4.

1. The cavity is dried with oil-free pressurized air.
2. The dentine is conditioned, then the adhesive is painted on to the dentine, following the manufacturer's instructions exactly. Any dentine adhesive spilt on to the enamel may need to be removed. Glass-ionomers bond to dentine and can be etched, making them very useful 'dentine adhesives' under composite.
3. The phosphoric acid etching gel is painted on to the enamel, coating the vertical enamel walls of the cavity and a 2 mm band of enamel surrounding the cavity. Etchant is available as a clear or coloured liquid or gel; a coloured gel is the easiest and safest to use. Phosphoric acid etchant must not contact the dentine, or it will reach and irritate the pulpal cells, so the dentine is protected before the enamel is etched. Even in a dead tooth, dentine cannot be etched, but the etchant is sometimes used as a dentine conditioner.

4. After 30–60 seconds, the etchant is rinsed off for 30–60 seconds (or as advised by the manufacturer). The gingivae, mucosae and tongue are protected to prevent burning with the acid.
5. The surface is dried with pressurized, oil-free air. Etched enamel has a frosted, matt appearance when dry. If this is not evident the etching procedure should be repeated. If fluoride has been applied to the enamel, this will impede the etching process. Any accidentally etched enamel will be remineralized in 2–3 days. It is essential that nothing touches the etched surface; all soft tissues, saliva and instruments must be kept out of the way. If the etched surface is touched, the exposed lattice will fill with the contaminating liquid or collapse when pressed; if this happens it should be re-etched.
6. The enamel-bonding agent (unfilled resin) is mixed (when necessary) and painted on to the etched enamel and the adhesive-coated dentine; the excess is blown off gently with oil-free pressurized air. The resin is cured, following the manufacturer's instructions.
7. The composite is mixed (for chemically

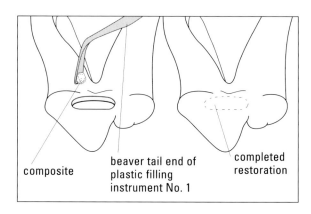

composite   beaver tail end of   completed
                 plastic filling   restoration
                 instrument No. 1

FIG. 6.4 Filling the prepared cavity of the early class V carious cavity of an upper fourth premolar shown in Fig. 6.3; labial aspect. Left: Placing composite in the prepared cavity. Right: Completed restoration.

cured composites) and placed in the cavity, overfilling the cavity and packing it well into the undercut and on to the etched enamel, using a plastic filling instrument. Over-use of instruments will introduce air bubbles into the restoration, so the composite is placed with minimal use of instruments. A 'composite syringe' may be used to inject the composite into the cavity; this minimizes the introduction of air bubbles into the composite. A piece of thin plastic kitchen wrap or a dental mylar strip can be placed over the composite, and the composite then compressed into the cavity; this prevents the composite from sticking to the instruments.

8. Chemically cured composite will cure in several minutes. Light-cured composite is cured incrementally, as the light can only penetrate effectively to a depth of 2 mm. If the cavity is deeper than 2 mm, a 2 mm depth of composite is packed into the base of the cavity and cured. Then another 2 mm depth of composite is added and cured, continuing in this fashion until the cavity is overfilled. Once the techniques are mastered, it is not necessary to overfill the cavity. If the cavity is filled with exactly the required amount of composite, the surface can be shaped well using a piece of thin, transparent plastic, through which it can then be cured. Very little finishing is then required.

9. The composite is shaped to recreate the tooth's normal anatomy and smoothed flush with the tooth surface, using a finishing bur (e.g. 7901).

10. When occlusal surfaces are filled, the occlusion must be checked, to ensure there are no high areas of the restoration which would interfere with the occlusion and cause pain. A length of articulating carbon ribbon is placed on the filling. The endotracheal tube is removed, the tongue placed in the mouth and the teeth closed firmly into occlusion. The endotracheal tube is reinserted and the surface of the filling examined for marks. Any high areas will be marked with the carbon, and are removed with a finishing bur.

11. The surface is finished with sanding discs, then rubber abrasives and finally polished with fine pumice in a rubber prophy cup.

12. A final lustre can be achieved by applying a thin coat of unfilled resin to the re-etched washed and dried finished composite surface.

A deep cavity

The procedure is illustrated in Fig. 6.5.

1. The prepared cavity is thoroughly washed, then dried with oil-free, pressurized air.

2. If the pulp has been exposed, an endodontic procedure is performed (e.g. direct pulp capping or root canal therapy). If the pulp is covered by less than 2 mm of dentine, it needs protection; indirect pulp capping is performed. Hard-setting calcium hydroxide cement is placed over the base of the cavity preparation to a depth of 1–2 mm. This should not extend up the walls of the cavity, unless a branch of the pulp chamber lies within 2 mm of a cavity wall (sometimes seen in deep occlusal lesions of the molars). It is preferable to leave a very thin layer of carious dentine over the pulp and to perform indirect pulp capping than to expose the pulp (see 'Pulp Capping', p. 73).

3. Once set, the excess calcium hydroxide is removed from the walls with a dental spoon excavator or a small, pear-shaped or round bur.

4. The cavity is flushed clean, and dried with pressurized, oil-free air. The dentine conditioner, for use prior to glass-ionomer application, is painted on to the cavity walls and floor, over both the dentine and the set calcium hydroxide cement. This conditioner is available as a clear or coloured liquid; the coloured is easier to use. The cavity is rinsed according to the manufacturer's instructions (after 10 or 30 seconds), then dried gently to leave a fine residue of moisture.

5. A layer of type II glass-ionomer cement is

placed on top of the calcium hydroxide. This further protects the pulp and provides strength to the base of the restoration, preventing the calcium hydroxide from being pushed into the pulp chamber. This layer can be almost as thick as the dentine (2–4 mm), but must not be less than 0.5 mm thick. There must be space for at least a 2 mm depth of composite to be placed on top. Plastic filling instruments may be used; PTFE- and titanium-coated instruments are available to minimize the difficulties encountered when glass-ionomer sticks to the metal instruments. The use of a composite syringe makes filling the cavity even easier. Faster setting type III cements are available for this technique but, as they are not as strong as type II cements, they are not recommended for use in animals. Where aesthetics are of prime importance, a tooth-coloured type II glass ionomer cement can be used. However, a reinforced type II cement (e.g. silver–cermet cement) is the strongest and is preferred for use in animals.

6. The glass-ionomer is allowed to set, following the manufacturer's instructions.

7. Excess glass-ionomer is removed from the enamel with a small pear-shaped or round bur, with water irrigation. Trimming the cement without water irrigation will dry it excessively, irreversibly damaging its surface. The surface is flushed clean, then dried with oil-free pressurized air.

8. The enamel (to 2 mm around the cavity margin) and glass-ionomer are coated with etching gel and etched for a maximum of 30 seconds. The surfaces are rinsed for at least 30 seconds, then dried thoroughly, with pressurized, oil-free air. It is essential that glass-ionomer is not etched for more than 30 seconds, or its surface will be irreparably damaged. The etched surfaces must not be contaminated.

9. The composite-bonding agent is mixed, applied to all the etched surfaces, and cured, following the manufacturer's instructions. It is important to apply and cure the bonding agent immediately after etching; this will protect the glass-ionomer from dehydration.

10. The composite is mixed (where necessary) and placed in the prepared site. Plastic filling instruments and composite syringes can be used. A minimum depth of 2 mm of composite is recommended.

11. The surface is finished as for the superficial cavity.

Using Amalgam

As amalgam does not stick to tooth structure,

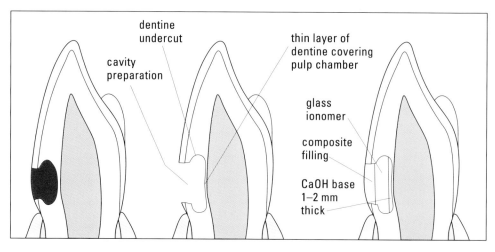

FIG. 6.5 The treatment of a deep class V lesion in a lower first molar; longitudinal section. Left: The carious lesion, separated from the pulp by a thin layer of dentine. Centre: The cavity preparation, not exposing the pulp. Right: The completed restoration.

it can be retained by the dentine undercut and an amalgam adhesive. The techniques for preparing the cavity and applying the amalgam adhesive are similar to those described under 'using composite'. The manufacturer's instructions must always be followed exactly as there are numerous small variations between products. The procedure for using amalgam to fill the cavity on top of the adhesive is as described below, the 'prepared cavity' being the cavity with the amalgam adhesive already in place. Without the use of an adhesive, the retention of the amalgam filling depends entirely on the dentine undercut, which has to be more severe, with the opening of the cavity significantly smaller than its base.

The techniques for filling both superficial and deep cavities with amalgam are the same as for composite, up to the point before the prepared cavity is etched. The surfaces are not etched when amalgam is used without an adhesive, but the cavity must be lined with a cavity liner (e.g. type III glass-ionomer or copalite cavity varnish, with or without fluoride) to prevent microleakage.

1. The amalgam alloy is mixed using the precapsulated forms, or in an amalgamator.
2. The mixed amalgam is transferred into an amalgam well or a dappen dish.
3. An amalgam-carrier is pressed into the amalgam, packing its hollow tip with amalgam.
4. A small amount of amalgam is placed in the prepared cavity and packed down with a flat-ended amalgam plugger (or condenser), pressing it into the cavity margins, ensuring no voids are left unfilled.
5. A little more amalgam is added and pressed into the cavity. This is repeated until the cavity is overfilled with amalgam.
6. The initial set takes 5–10 minutes, during which the amalgam is carved.
7. The amalgam is carved to shape, with repeated, light, carving strokes, using an amalgam carver. The amalgam is carved along the cavity margin or from tooth surface to alloy; working from alloy to tooth creates ledging.

8. When occlusal surfaces are filled, the occlusion must be checked, to ensure that there are no high areas of the restoration which would interfere with the occlusion and cause pain. A length of articulating carbon ribbon is placed on the filling. The endotracheal tube is removed, the tongue placed in the mouth and the teeth closed firmly into occlusion. The endotracheal tube is reinserted and the surface of the filling examined for marks. Any high areas will be marked with the carbon, and are removed with the amalgam carver or a finishing bur. The filling is burnished with a ball- or pear-ended burnisher.
9. The final set of the amalgam is completed after 24 hours, so the surface cannot be polished to a shine until then.
10. A large cutting bur can be used to reshape the restoration at this stage, if necessary.
11. The surface is burnished and polished with abrasive points and paste. Omitting this polishing step leaves the surface of the amalgam filling rough enough for plaque and debris to adhere easily. It is therefore essential that the amalgam filling is properly finished the day after its insertion. As this requires another anaesthetic, it is a serious diadvantage to the use of amalgam in animals.

Using Glass-Ionomers

Glass-ionomers can be used as cavity liners under composite or amalgam or for the entire filling of non-occlusal cavities, for example feline subgingival resorptive lesions (see below). Some manufacturers suggest that no conditioning of the tooth surface is required. Better results are generally obtained if a tooth surface conditioner is used.

Feline subgingival resorptive lesions

The restoration of a Class II feline subgingival resorptive lesion is illustrated in Fig. 6.6.

1. A thorough scale and polish is performed on all the teeth. The lesion is detected and

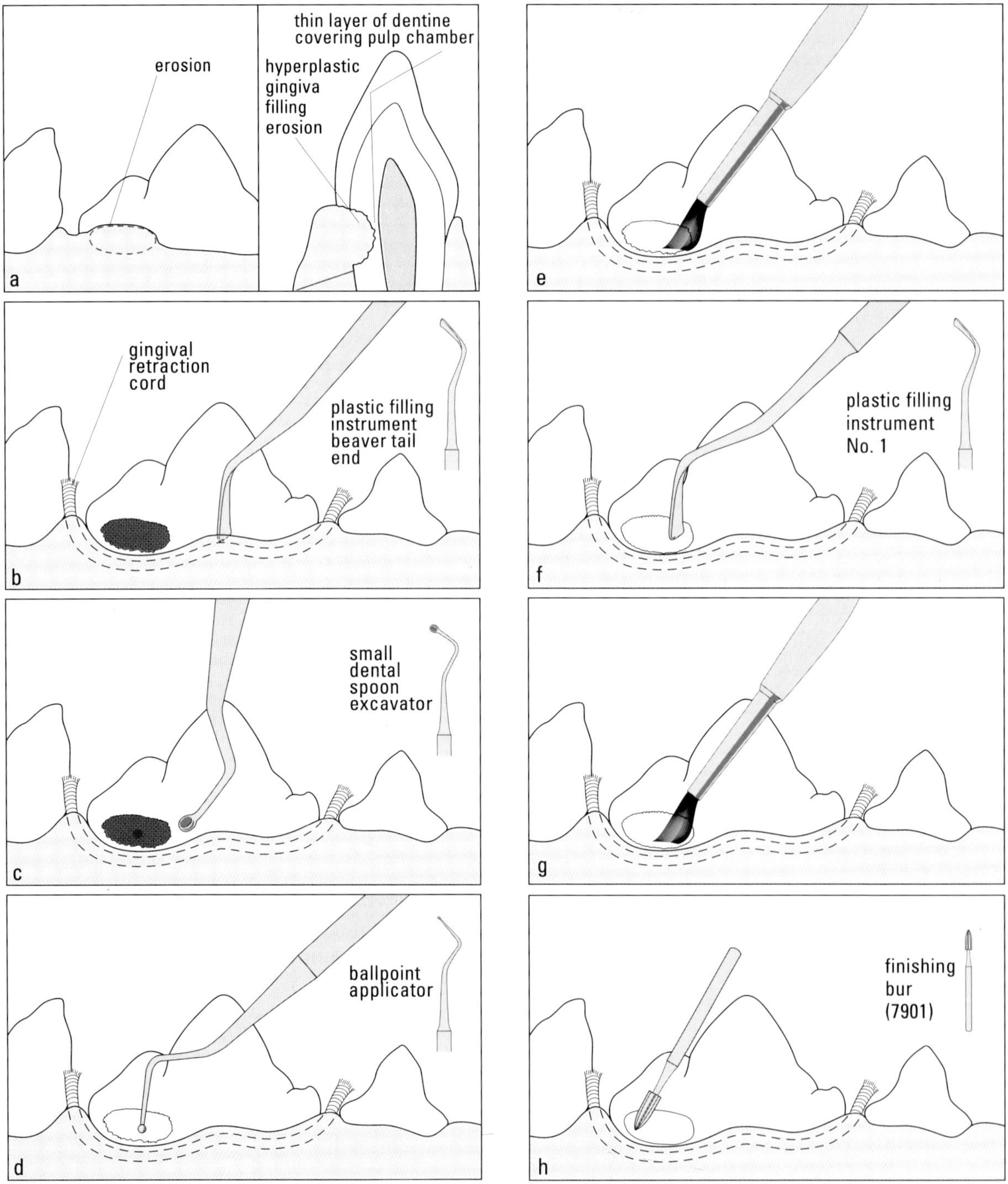

Fig. 6.6 The restoration of a feline subgingival resorptive lesion in the lower second premolar. (a) The gingiva covering the erosion. Inset: Section of the tooth showing the extent of the lesion, not exposing the pulp, and the incision line for the removal of the hyperplastic gingiva. (b) Inserting the gingival retraction cord. (c) Excavating any debris. (d) Placing calcium hydroxide cement over the thin layer of dentine. (e) Cleaning the surface with conditioner. (f) Overfilling the prepared cavity with glass-ionomer. (g) Applying varnish over the setting glass-ionomer. (h) Shaping the restoration and removing excess glass-ionomer.

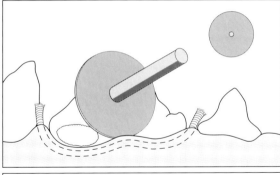
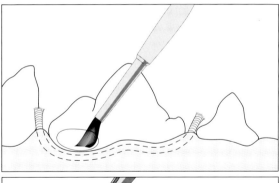
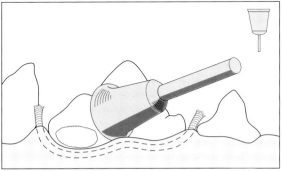
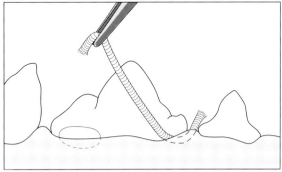

Fig.6.6 (continued) (i) Smoothing the filling with sanding discs. (j) Finishing the restoration with rubber abrasives. (k) Applying varnish to the finished restoration. (l) Removing the gingival retraction cord.

explored using a Shepherd's hook explorer.

2. Radiographs are taken and the lesion classified.

3. The hyperplastic gingival tissue is cut with a bevelled edge, using a scalpel or electrosurgery and recreating the normal anatomical features. At least 2 mm of attached gingiva must be left (see Fig. 5.13). If electrosurgery is used, it eliminates haemorrhage, leaving a dry field. Retraction cord will probably not be necessary, but an allowance must be made for the 1 mm slough which usually follows the use of heat for cutting.

4. The gingiva is lifted out of the lesion and, if necessary, a gingival retraction cord packed deep into the gingival crevice with the flat, beaver-tail end of a plastic filling instrument No. 1. It is important that none of the cord impinges on the cavity. This will control the haemorrhage and encourage the gingiva to retract. If necessary, gingival retraction liquid can be dropped on to the area to help with haemostasis. The gingiva must be moved apically far enough to expose the lesion; it may be necessary to raise a flap, as described in Chapters 5 and 8.

5. The debris is removed from the cavity with a dental spoon excavator, and flushed away with pressurized water. The cavity is dried with oil-free, pressurized air. The proximity of the pulp is estimated. If the pulp is visible through a thin layer of dentine, indirect pulp capping is performed. If the erosion has entered the pulp chamber, exposing the pulp, the tooth should be extracted; direct pulp capping is not applicable because gingival granulation tissue will have invaded the pulp chamber, and 'granulation tissue capping' will fail.

6. Hard-setting calcium hydroxide cement is mixed and placed over the thin layer of dentine covering the pulp chamber (indirect pulp capping). Excess cement is removed with the dental spoon excavator and

the cavity flushed clean, then dried.

7. Tooth surface conditioner (25% polyacrylic acid) is brushed into the lesion. This conditions the surface, removing any organic debris and opening the dentinal tubules. It is available as a coloured or clear liquid; the coloured is easier to use. After the recommended time (usually 10–15 seconds), the conditioner is thoroughly washed off. The prepared cavity is then partially dried, with pressurized, oil-free air, to leave a slight residual dampness in the cavity.

8. The glass-ionomer is mixed exactly following the manufacturer's instructions. A reinforced type II glass-ionomer is recommended (e.g. the silver–cermet–cements), although if appearance is of great importance, an aesthetic, tooth-coloured type II can be used. Mixing on a cold glass slab will slow the setting time, giving a little extra working time (this is very useful when one is learning the technique). The use of a light-cured glass-ionomer will provide as much working time as is needed as it can be cured exactly when required; this is a much more convenient and versatile setting mechanism. The glass-ionomer is placed in the prepared cavity. Plastic filling instruments may be used; PTFE- or titanium coated and plastic instruments are available to minimize the difficulties encountered when glass-ionomer sticks to the metal instruments. The use of a composite syringe to inject glass ionomer into the cavity makes successful filling of the cavity even easier, enabling all the voids to be filled whilst minimizing the introduction of air bubbles. The material is pressed firmly into the cavity to fill all the recesses. The cavity is overfilled, glass-ionomer protruding beyond the margins of the cavity.

9. Immediately after placing the material, varnish is brushed on to the setting glass-ionomer, following the manufacturer's instructions, to protect it from dehydration. If this is neglected, the material will crack and fail. As an alternative to the varnish, a piece of thin plastic sheet (e.g. kitchen wrap) can be placed over the filling and pressed gently to the correct shape. The glass-ionomer is light-cured or left to set, then the plastic sheet is removed. Any interference during the setting time will interfere with the setting reaction, destroying the initial bond formation; the filling will then fall out.

10. After setting, the restoration is shaped using a 12-bladed finishing bur at high speed with water irrigation (unless the manufacturers recommend a different method), or a finishing diamond bur at low speed. The restoration should be shaped to recreate the natural anatomy as far as possible. There must be no step or gap between the restoration and the tooth surface; this junction must be smooth.

11. Fine-grade sanding discs are used at low speed to shape and smooth the restoration, taking care not to overheat the tooth.

12. Abrasive rubber cups followed by the prophy cup and prophy paste are used to polish the surface.

13. The restoration is rinsed, dried and coated with varnish or unfilled composite resin after etching (see 'Using Composite').

14. The gingival retraction cord is removed and the whole area rinsed and dried.

15. It is wise to apply a fluoride or foam varnish to all the teeth, above and below the gingiva. Fluoride is thought to harden the enamel and dentine, to reduce sensitivity, to have antibacterial properties and, possibly, to reduce the progress of these resorptive lesions.

Enamel Dysplasia and Staining

Dysplasia and staining of the enamel are common conditions, particularly in dogs. Enamel dysplasia is the defective or incomplete formation of enamel. It may be hereditary, in which case the temporary and permanent dentition are affected, or it may be environmental (e.g. local injury or infection, fever, nutritional deficiencies, ingestion of chemicals such as excess fluoride) involving either dentition and sometimes only one tooth. Dysplasia results if the insult occurs during the formation of the enamel, amelogenesis. When affected teeth erupt, their enamel may be visibly discoloured in patches or partly missing, or it may appear normal, then discolour, absorbing colour from food, or flake off later. The clinical significance of enamel dysplasia is that exposed dentine is painful. These lesions become less painful as the animal ages when secondary dentine is laid down by the odontoblasts lining the pulp cavity. The dentine also thickens during the development of normal teeth.

Stained enamel secondary to the administration of tetracycline during amelogenesis in an immature animal is unlikely to be weak, but may be considered aesthetically unpleasant.

It is important to check the occlusion before embarking on a repair, to ensure that there is space for the restoration. The stained or damaged enamel is removed, removing as little tooth structure as possible. Minor undercuts are made around the cavity. Additional retention may be attained by drilling two or three tiny holes 0.5 mm deep in the dentine, on opposite sides of the cavity. Any exposed dentine is coated with a thin layer of tooth-coloured glass-ionomer or a dentine adhesive. The cavity is then acid etched and filled with composite in the same way as for a superficial caries lesion. It is important that the restoration is not too bulky and that it does not interfere with the occlusion.

7
Endodontics

Endodontics is the treatment of the pulp of a tooth. Inflamed or necrotic pulp is removed (pulpectomy) and the root canal cleaned and filled. Exposed but healthy pulp may be saved by performing a vital pulpotomy with direct pulp capping. Pulp which is almost exposed, but is still protected by a thin layer of dentine, is treated with indirect pulp capping. In this way, teeth damaged so severely that the pulp is involved can be saved and do not have to be extracted. This prevents the possible post-extraction complications of oronasal fistula formation, pain, tongue protrusion, dysphagia and bony deformity. Endodontic therapy is the least traumatic means of treating a tooth with pulpal involvement. Once the techniques are mastered, endodontic therapy is also the easiest, the safest and the quickest method.

Aetiology of Pulpal Pathology

The pulp may be involved in the following ways.

Damage to the Tooth Crown, Exposing Pulp

The tooth may be damaged and the pulp exposed by trauma, attrition, carious decay, feline subgingival dental resorption or tooth shortening. This form of damage is particularly common in cats after accidents and fights, and in dogs after accidents, fights, catching stones and chewing bones and bricks.

Disruption of the Apical Blood Supply

If a tooth is hit, but not so hard that it fractures, it may move far enough to disrupt its apical blood supply. The pulp dies and the breakdown products of the blood diffuse into the dentinal tubules. The 'bruise' colour is clearly visible through the enamel. The necrotic pulp causes an inflammatory reaction around the apex of the tooth. This periapical lesion may be a granuloma, cyst or an abscess. An abscess is very painful and is a common sequel to an apical cyst or granuloma. Even if it is thought that an abscess has not yet formed, the tooth should be treated endodontically to prevent the formation of an abscess.

Caries

By the time a carious lesion in a tooth is noticed, it has often progressed through the enamel and dentine and has encroached upon the pulp. There may be a thin layer of sclerotic, secondary dentine protecting the pulp, but this may be breached by overzealous cavity preparation or the continuation of the process of decay.

Feline Subgingival Resorptive Lesions

These lesions commonly involve the pulp chamber. It is rarely possible to save teeth which have suffered such a degree of resorption, as the tooth structure is so severely weakened. Canine teeth can often be treated, but for affected premolars, molars and incisors, extraction is usually the only treatment once the pulp is involved. Treatment prior to this stage is covered in Chapter 6.

Thermal Damage

Thermal injury to the pulp is usually iatrogenic. Teeth can easily be overheated to the extent that the pulp is damaged by, for example: poor polishing technique, using too much pressure, too little prophy paste, too many rpm or failing to move the prophy cup continuously over the tooth surface; poor mechanical scaling technique, using insufficient cooling water, too much pressure or failing to move the scaling tip continuously over the tooth surface; or careless use of thermocautery, diathermy or electrosurgery units near the teeth. The pulp dies, the tooth becomes discoloured and a periapical lesion forms.

Haematogenous Spread of Infection

Necrotic pulp is more susceptible to haematogenous spread of infection than is healthy pulp, although both are thought to become infected by this route.

Pathogenesis of Pulpal Pathology

An open pulp chamber allows bacteria into the root canal system of a tooth. The pulp becomes inflamed and eventually necrotic. This pulpal pathology frequently extends into the periapical tissues, producing a periapical lesion visible radiographically as an 'apical halo'. The lesion may be a granuloma, a cyst or an abscess. The granulomas and cysts usually become abscesses eventually. The abscess forms fistulous tracts which eventually emerge as discharging sinuses either extra- or intraorally ('gum boil'), or as subcutaneous swellings (commonly infraorbital or submaxillary abscesses).

Damaged pulp becomes inflamed. Without an opening through the enamel and dentine through which they can escape, the breakdown products of the inflamed pulp pass into the horizontal tubules of the dentine and are visible through the enamel as a pinkish purple discoloration. As the pulp becomes necrotic, so the colour turns more grey and periapical pathology develops as described above.

Clinical Signs and Diagnosis

Initially, these conditions are extremely painful, as the pulpal nerves are exposed or inflamed and irritated. If it is left untreated, the pulp becomes infected and necrotic. The sen-

sation of pain ceases once the pulp has become totally necrotic, but soon returns when an apical abscess develops. When the abscess discharges its contents through an intra- or extraoral sinus, the pressure is relieved and the pain subsides. As with any chronic infection, this is a generally debilitating condition.

Animals seem to be particularly tolerant of pain and often show few clinical signs. The following symptoms may be noticed:

- haemorrhage from a recently fractured tooth
- tooth discoloration: pink to purple to grey indicates pulpal pathology; yellowish brown discoloration is due either to enamel dysplasia or to the administration of tetracycline whilst the enamel is forming (which usually involves more than one tooth)
- a black spot on a fractured or worn crown, without caries: if a sharp explorer passes into the black area, the pulp is involved; if the spot is smooth and impenetrable, it is probably the dark brown, secondary, reparative dentine produced as a result of excessive attrition, which needs no endodontic treatment
- facial swelling: this is often an infraorbital abscess, which generally indicates the presence of a periapical abscess of the upper fourth premolar, usually the result of a coronal slab fracture with pulpal exposure
- a discharging sinus, through the gingiva, the mucosa or the skin, suggesting apical abscessation.

Other symptoms include: tooth sensitivity and 'mouth shyness'; unwillingness to bite hard (particularly noticeable in working dogs); dysphagia avoiding hard food, chewing on one side; excessive salivation; jaw chattering, constant licking; reluctance to carry sticks or newspapers; general malaise; premature ageing, which should disappear after successful treatment of the dental lesion; disinterest in play; and evidence of an acute or chronic infection; and symptoms as diverse as infertility and aggression.

Radiography is essential to identify the affected tooth, to discover the extent of the damage and to assess the periapical pathology.

Treatment

There are three pulpal treatments, each of which has specific indications. They are pulp capping, vital pulpotomy and root canal therapy.

Pulp Capping

Indications

Pulp capping is the most minor pulp treatment. A small pulpal exposure created by the removal of excess dentine during the preparation of a cavity can be treated by direct pulp capping provided the pulp has not been grossly contaminated. If the pulp is visible through a thin layer of normal, sclerotic (reparative) or carious dentine, but is not actually exposed, it needs to be protected from the final filling material and stimulated to thicken and repair by indirect pulp capping. Provided the surrounding dentine is healthy, the thin layer of carious dentine need not be removed. It is better to avoid a pulpal exposure where possible.

Calcium hydroxide is used to stimulate the dentine to repair, producing secondary, reparative dentine under the carious dentine; it also has some antibacterial activity. Glass-ionomers contain flouride, so lining the cavity with a glass-ionomer base allows fluoride to leach out into the surrounding dentine. Fluoride is cariostatic, reduces the sensitivity of exposed dentine, strengthens dentine and is antibacterial, and thus the condition of the cavity improves. Glass-ionomers are also biocompatible and bond into the dentine, improving its strength.

Equipment

Paper points (rolled absorbent paper)
Calcium hydroxide powder
Calcium hydroxide hard-setting cement
Mixing slab
Mixing spatula
Ballpoint applicator
Small sharp dental spoon excavator
High-speed handpiece (low-speed will suffice if high-speed is not available)
Pear-shaped bur size 330
Glass-ionomer or zinc oxide and eugenol hard-setting base cement
Final filling material with the recommended tooth surface preparing agents
Plastic filling instrument PFI No. 1
Finishing bur size 7901
Green then white finishing abrasive rubber wheels, cups or stones; or fine-grade sanding discs for finishing
Antibiotics

Procedures

Direct pulp capping

1. An injection of antibiotic may be given as soon as an accidental exposure is made. The freshly exposed pulp bleeds and this helps to flush out any contaminants. The cavity is flushed gently with sterile water until all the debris is removed.

2. Haemorrhage is controlled by gently pressing the blunt ends of large, sterile paper points on to the pulp. Continuous, gentle pressure is applied for 3–5 minutes to encourage clotting. Sterile cotton wool dampened with sterile saline may also be used to control haemorrhage but care must be taken not to leave any threads of cotton wool in the canal afterwards. A little adrenaline (epinephrine) may be applied on a paper point to aid haemorrhage control if all other methods fail. Caustic or thermal cautery is never used to control pulpal haemorrhage as it is far too damaging to the pulp.

3. Pressurized, oil-free air is used to dry the cavity.

4. A little calcium hydroxide powder is applied and gently pressed on to the pulp with the blunt end of a sterile paper point; this absorbs any remaining blood. The excess powder is removed with a dental spoon excavator, levelling the base of the cavity, and the cavity scraped clean. Hard-setting calcium hydroxide cement is mixed on a mixing pad or glass slab. With a ballpoint applicator, the cement is placed carefully over the exposure and the adjacent

dentine. The cement should not be spread up the sides of the cavity, unless an exposure or a near exposure involves the cavity wall. After it has set hard, any excess cement is removed from the cavity walls with a dental spoon excavator or, very carefully, with a pear-shaped bur. Calcium hydroxide powder is now in direct contact with the pulp; the cement seals the exposure and any areas of thin dentine. In some circumstances, the cement may be placed in direct contact with the pulp.

5. The cavity is lined with a material to impart strength to the base of the restoration, preventing the cement from being pushed into the pulp. This also provides a further barrier between the pulp and the final filling, protecting the pulp from thermal insult and chemical leakage. The two materials most commonly used are glass-ionomer or zinc oxide and eugenol (ZnOE) base cement. Glass-ionomer is the easiest to use as it is compatible with all final filling materials and bonds to dentine and enamel, whereas ZnOE prevents composite from setting and binds with nothing. As glass-ionomer also leaches fluoride into the surrounding dentine and enamel, it is now the material of choice.

    The tooth surface is prepared exactly following the manufacturer's instructions. The material is mixed and applied to the base of the cavity over the calcium hydroxide cement and on to the surrounding dentine. Thus, the base and part of the walls of the cavity are coated in glass-ionomer or ZnOE, completely sealing the pulp chamber. If glass-ionomer is used as the liner, the entire dentine surface is coated with it.

6. The final filling material is selected (see Chapter 6). The cavity surface (lined and bare) is prepared according to the manufacturer's instructions. If compatible products are chosen to line and fill the cavity, the procedure is somewhat simplified and the results more reliable. The cavity is filled, finished and polished.

Indirect pulp capping

1. The cavity is flushed clean with pressurized water and dried with pressurized, oil-free air.
2. Hard-setting calcium hydroxide cement is mixed and placed over the thin area of dentine, extending on to normal dentine, as in Step 4 for the direct pulp capping procedure. Any excess is removed with a dental spoon excavator or a bur.
3. The procedure continues from Step 5 of direct pulp capping, above.

Six months post-operatively, the cavity may be reopened to remove any remaining caries over the newly formed dentine bridge, but this step is not usually necessary. If it is done, the cavity is then lined with glass-ionomer and filled.

Vital Pulpotomy

Indications

Vital pulpotomy is the treatment of choice when treating healthy, freshly exposed pulp in immature animals where the root apex is still open and the dentine wall is thin. The remaining treated vital pulp will continue to produce dentine, lengthening the root (apexogenesis), closing the apex (apexification) and thickening the dentine wall. Following the removal of the coronal pulp, the remaining healthy pulp is encouraged to produce a secondary dentine bridge by treating it with calcium hydroxide. This is rarely the technique of choice for mature animals with closed apices and thick dentine walls, unless performed under sterile conditions as a disarming procedure.

If the pulp is treated within one hour of accidental exposure, whilst inflammation and infection are minimal, the prognosis is good. The longer the pulp has been exposed, the poorer the prognosis. The health of the pulp can be assessed by the colour and flow of the pulpal blood on excising the coronal 5–8 mm of pulp; bright, red, free-flowing haemorrhage suggests healthy pulpal tissue. This is a very subjective assessment and should be used with caution. It is a helpful guide in situations where the time of the exposure is unknown.

Surgical crown height reduction is a sterile procedure, which should prevent infection of the pulp. The procedure is usually limited to the canine teeth, where it may be used to treat traumatic malocclusions (e.g. medially displaced lower canines impinging on the hard palate) or as a disarming technique (e.g. for overzealous sheep-dogs, where it is thought the dog is damaging the sheep by biting too hard).

Equipment

All the equipment which may contact the pulp must be sterile, marked *.

High-speed handpiece (low-speed will suffice if high-speed is not available)
* Cooling water or saline from a syringe if it is not available through the handpiece
* Tapered fissure bur size 699 or 700; a safe-sided diamond disc is not recommended
* Gauze swabs or cotton wool
* Paper points
* Round-headed bur size 2 or 4; or pear-shaped bur size 331 or 332
* Small sharp dental spoon excavator
* Calcium hydroxide powder
* Plastic filling instrument
Calcium hydroxide hard-setting cement
Mixing slab
Mixing spatula
Ballpoint applicator
Pear-shaped bur size 330
Glass-ionomer or composite filling material with the recommended tooth surface preparing agents
Finishing bur size 7901
Green then white finishing abrasive rubber wheels, cups or stones; or fine-grade sanding discs for finishing
Antibiotics
Radiographic equipment

Procedure

The procedure is illustrated in Fig. 7.1.
1. An antibiotic is given by injection. A radiograph is taken to check for additional fractures and other complicating factors. The teeth are thoroughly cleaned. The affected tooth is prepared for sterile surgery.

2. If canine crown height is to be reduced, a sterile tapered fissure bur (or a safe-sided diamond disc, with care) is used with sterile water coolant to cut through the tooth, at 90° to the long axis of the tooth, at the same height as the lateral incisors (Fig. 7.1a).
3. If the pulp has been exposed traumatically, any jagged edges are removed with a tapered fissure bur. Access to the pulp chamber may be enlarged if necessary with a sterile round bur.
4. The coronal 5–8 mm of pulp is amputated as atraumatically as possible, under sterile conditions, to remove any infected pulp and create space for the medicaments to treat and protect the pulp. The aim is to reach healthy pulpal tissue while minimizing damage to it. This can be achieved in one of three ways (Fig. 7.1b).

Either

A sharp, sterile spoon excavator is inserted between the pulp and the dentine wall to a depth of 5–8 mm. It is turned into the pulp and withdrawn with the coronal portion of pulp.

Or

A new, sharp, sterile round bur in the straight, slow-speed handpiece with sterile water or saline irrigation is used to cut through the coronal 5–8 mm of pulp. These burs are long, allowing the removal of more pulp if necessary. The sterile irrigating fluid is delivered from a syringe on to the cutting bur. This provides two advantages when compared with using high-speed:
• the drill's cooling water system does not need to be sterilized;
• the fluid is dribbled from the syringe, rather than being delivered under pressure from the high-speed handpiece right onto the pulp.
It is essential to use a new, sharp bur to ensure the pulp is cut rather than twisted and pulled.

Or

A sharp, sterile, round bur with sterile water coolant, in the high-speed handpiece, is inserted into the pulp chamber, cutting through the coronal pulp to a depth of 5–8 mm. At high speed, a sharp bur cuts the tissue without tearing or twisting it and so is thought to be almost as atraumatic as cutting with a dental spoon excavator. High-speed burs are shorter than straight burs for the straight, slow-speed handpiece, which may prevent the removal of sufficient pulp. Care should be taken to avoid pushing dentine or dentinal shavings on to the

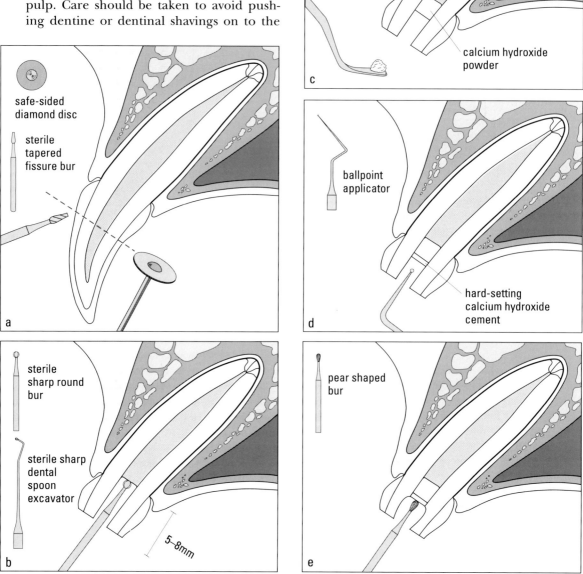

Fig. 7.1 Tooth shortening and vital pulpotomy on a mature upper canine tooth. (a) Reducing the height of the canine. (b) Amputating the coronal 5–8 mm of pulp. (c) Placing the calcium hydroxide powder. (d) Placing the hard-setting calcium hydroxide cement. (e) Making the undercut in the dentine.

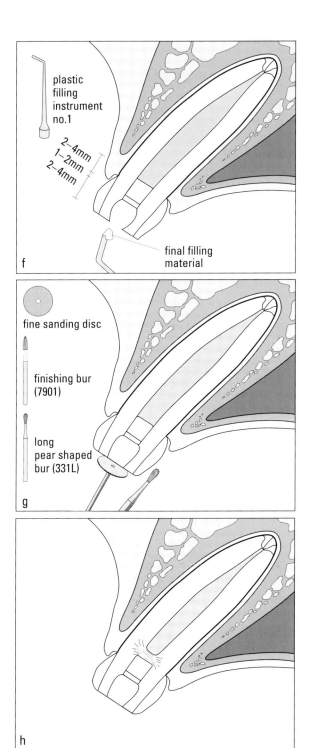

plastic filling instrument no.1

2–4mm
1–2mm
2–4mm

final filling material

f

fine sanding disc

finishing bur (7901)

long pear shaped bur (331L)

g

h

FIG. 7.1 (continued) Tooth shortening and vital pulpotomy on a mature upper canine tooth. (f) Inserting the final filling material. (g) Shaping and finishing the restoration. (h) Dentine bridge formation and thickening of the dentine wall.

pulp as this will increase pulpal haemorrhage.

5. Haemorrhage is controlled by inserting the blunt ends of large, sterile paper points into the canal and gently pressing them on to the pulp. The paper points should not be continually removed and reinserted, but continuous, gentle pressure should be applied for 3–5 minutes to encourage clotting. Sterile cotton wool dampened with sterile saline may also be used to control haemorrhage; care must be taken not to leave any threads of cotton wool in the canal afterwards. A small amount of adrenaline (epinephrine) may be applied on the blunt end of a paper point to help control haemorrhage. Caustic or thermal cautery is never used to control haemorrhage, as it is far too damaging to the pulp.

Healthy pulp usually stops bleeding after 5 minutes. Haemorrhage continuing beyond this time usually indicates the presence of inflamed pulp; this must be removed, so another 1–2 mm of pulp is amputated. If haemorrhage is still uncontrolled after a further 5 minutes of continuous pressure, another 1–2 mm of pulp is amputated. If this fails to control the haemorrhage, the pulp should be removed and a conventional root canal treatment performed.

6. Calcium hydroxide powder is placed directly on to the pulp (Fig. 7.1c). This will also control any residual minor haemorrhage. The powder is carried to the area on a sterile plastic filling instrument (beaver-tail) or in a metal amalgam carrier and inserted in small increments into the pulp chamber with the blunt end of a sterile paper point. It is gently packed on to the pulp. A blunt, broad-ended endodontic plugger or the rounded end of the plastic filling instrument is used gently to compress the powder on to the pulp to a final depth of 2–4 mm.

7. A hard-setting calcium hydroxide cement is mixed and placed on top of the calcium hydroxide powder with a ballpoint

applicator, to a depth of 1–2 mm (Fig. 7.1d). This provides additional protection and insulation of the pulp and lends some strength to the base of the restoration. A zinc oxide and eugenol base may be used instead of the calcium hydroxide paste, but it is incompatible with composite filling materials.

8. A pear-shaped bur, size 330, is used to clean the remaining 2–4 mm of pulp chamber walls, removing excess cement and debris (Fig. 7.1e). An undercut is made to create a retentive shelf for the final filling. As little dentine as possible should be removed when making the undercut so as to minimize the weakening of the tooth. The site is flushed with pressurized water and dried with oil-free air.

9. A glass-ionomer or composite is used to fill the prepared site. The manufacturer's instructions should be followed exactly in preparing the tooth surface and mixing the materials. Using the rounded end of the plastic filling instrument, the material is packed into the prepared site (Fig. 7.1f). It is essential that the material is tightly adapted to the cavity walls and that no air bubbles are introduced into the material during either mixing or placement. This will reduce the risks of microleakage which might otherwise allow bacteria and other contaminants to invade the pulp and produce pulpal infection.

10. Any rough tooth edges are smoothed with a long pear-shaped bur, size 331L. The restorative material and tooth margins are then smoothed with a finishing bur (e.g. 7901), followed by rubber abrasive polishing wheels (green then white) or fine sanding discs (Fig. 7.1g). When working across the tooth-filling margin, the instrument should always be moved towards the tooth surface to avoid pulling the filling away from the tooth margin. Final polishing is achieved with a prophy cup and prophy paste.

11. A radiograph is taken on completion for comparison with one to be taken later.

12. A 7–10 day course of antibiotics is advisable post-operatively.

13. A follow-up radiograph is taken 4-6 months after the operation, and compared with that taken immediately after the operation. The dentine wall should be thicker, the apex closed and the dentine bridge formed (Fig. 7.1h). If no dentine bridge is visible, and there are no signs of pulpal pathology (e.g. apical rarefaction, tooth discoloration), a third radiograph is taken 6 months later. If there are still no signs of dentine bridge formation, it is likely that the procedure has failed and a conventional root canal treatment is required. The apex should be examined closely for apical rarefaction indicative of apical pathology. Comparison with a radiograph of that animal's normal canine will help. When the technique is sucessful in young animals, a good dentine bridge can usually be detected 4 months post-operatively. Failure of the technique in young teeth is often dramatic. The large volume of necrotic pulp produces a large periapical lesion, easily visible radiographically, with discharging sinuses either through the skin or gingiva.

Root Canal Therapy

Indications

Irreversible pulpal pathology, pulpal damage and pulpal exposure in a mature animal are the indications for root canal therapy. The clinical appearance of these problems was described at the beginning of this chapter.

Severe damage to the pulp of an immature animal, if left untreated, will result in the situation where the dead pulp will not produce dentine, so the mature animal will have a tooth that is not fully developed, with thin dentine and possibly an open apex. Immature teeth can be treated if the pulp is irreparably damaged and the apex is open, using calcium hydroxide to fill the root canal. This stimulates a cementodentinal closure of the apex and is described after root canal therapy.

In animals, a discharging sinus or an apical abscess is usually resolved by the removal of the source of infection, the necrotic pulp, with conventional root canal treatment; it is rarely necessary to perform an apicectomy (a surgical root canal, where the apex is approached and sealed via a gingival or skin incision).

Equipment

High-speed handpiece (low-speed will suffice if high-speed is not available)

Burs: round-headed size 2, pear-shaped size 330 or 331

Barbed broaches: 25–30 mm 'human' lengths and 45–50 mm veterinary lengths

Root canal files: K-files and Hedstrom files in 25–30 mm 'human' lengths and 55–60 mm veterinary lengths, all in sizes 15–80; sizes 8, 10 and 90-140 are useful in 'human' lengths

Chelating agent: this is a paste which aids the debridement of the canal, softens the dentine and lubricates the canal, sometimes called 'root canal preparing agent'

Flushing solutions: sodium hypochlorite (bleach), hydrogen peroxide and sterile water in three separate 20 ml syringes

Pressurized air

Locking dental pliers or forceps (for placing paper points and gutta percha)

Paper points: assorted sizes in 'human' lengths and veterinary lengths

Gutta percha (GP): assorted sizes in 'human' lengths and veterinary lengths (this is a type of rubber; it melts in heat and is dissolved in chloroform)

Root canal filling cement: zinc oxide (powder) and eugenol (liquid), or Sealapex (a slow-setting calcium hydroxide paste)

Mixing slab

Mixing spatula

Spiral paste fillers: assorted sizes in 'human' length spiral paste fillers and lentulo spirals in 45–60 mm veterinary lengths

Low-speed contra-angle handpiece

Root canal explorer

Endodontic plugger

Spreader: gutta percha expander

Scalpel blade

Plastic filling instrument (PFI) No. 1 (metal, with beaver tail at one end and burnisher at the other); PFIs are also available in acrylic, for use with composite

Radiographic equipment

Calcium hydroxide hard-setting cement (if using zinc oxide and eugenol cement and composite)

Ballpoint applicator

Final filling material (composite, glass-ionomer or amalgam) with the recommended tooth surface preparing agents

Finishing bur (e.g. size 7901)

Green then white finishing abrasive rubber wheels, cups or stones: or fine-grade sanding discs for finishing

Antibiotics

Procedure

The objectives of root canal treatment are a clean canal, an apical seal and a sealed access.

1. The tooth is radiographed to ensure there are no complicating factors, which may favour a different procedure. The radiograph also helps to locate the apex exactly. The mouth is cleaned with chlorhexidene or povidone–iodine, paying particular attention to the affected tooth.

2. If there is no fracture of the crown through which the pulp chamber can be entered and the apex reached, an access is made through the crown into the pulp chamber. The access hole is made as small as possible, to minimize any further weakening of an already weakened tooth; however, it must be large enough to accommodate the file shafts, otherwise a false sensation of reaching the apical stop may be encountered due to a file shaft becoming jammed in the access hole. The access hole is drilled to point directly to the apex. There is usually a palpable bony prominence over the root of a tooth, leading to easy identification of the apex. A round (size 1 or 2) or pear-shaped (size 330 or 331) bur is used to make the access. When

drilling into enamel, the initial 0.5 mm depth is cut at 90° to the surface; the drill is then angled towards the apex. This reduces the risks of slipping whilst starting the cut. The hole is drilled directly over the pulp chamber as follows (Fig. 7.2).

Canine (Fig. 7.2a). On the rostral surface, 2 mm coronal to the gingival margin, drill into the pulp chamber, starting at 90° to the enamel surface, then turning to point the bur at the apex and the pulp chamber (which runs down the centre of the tooth). The apex of a dog's canine tooth lies apical to the rostral root of the second premolar.

Incisor (Fig. 7.2b). On the rostral surface, halfway down the crown, drill into the pulp chamber, starting at 90° to the enamel surface, then turning to point the bur at the apex and the pulp chamber (which runs down the centre of the tooth). These are small teeth, with small pulp chambers, so it may be necessary to use a smaller bur (round, size $\frac{1}{2}$)

It may be possible to make the access into the pulp chamber of the central incisors on the caudal (lingual) aspect, drilling almost vertically at the level of the cingulum (Fig. 7.2c). Flexible K-files are used to clean these root canals, as the access cannot point directly at the apex.

Multi-rooted teeth. The access holes are drilled directly over the root canal of each root. Previously, one huge access hole was drilled

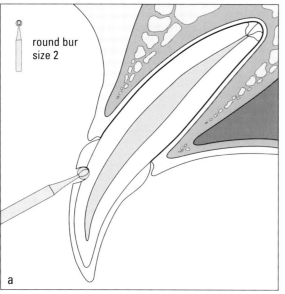

round bur
size 2

a

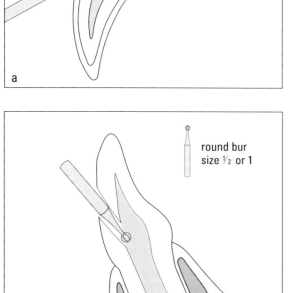

round bur
size ½ or 1

b

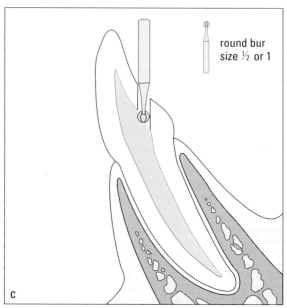

round bur
size ½ or 1

c

FIG. 7.2 Routes of access to the pulp chamber. (a) Access to the pulp chamber in an upper canine. (b) Access to the pulp chamber in a lower lateral incisor. (c) Access to the pulp chamber in a lower central incisor.

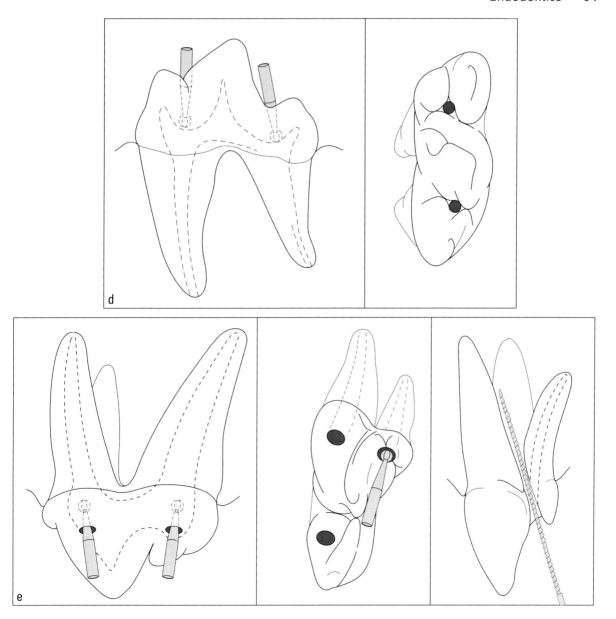

FIG. 7.2 (continued) Routes of access to the pulp chamber. (d) Access to the pulp chamber in a lower first molar: lateral aspect (left); dorsal aspect (right). (e) Access to the pulp chamber in an upper fourth premolar: lateral aspect (left); dorsal aspect (centre); a common error (right).

in the lateral wall of the tooth, from which all the root canals could be reached, with flexible files. This seriously weakens the crown and is not the preferred method. Access to the pulp chambers of the upper fourth premolar and the lower first molar of the dog are illustrated in Figs 7.2d and e.

The palatal root of the upper fourth premolar is small and tends to flare out medially. It is easy to drill the access for this root into the furcation (Fig. 7.2e). Direct the bur towards the apex (medially in this case) and stop drilling as soon as the pulp chamber is reached. Gentle exploration with a 25 mm size 10 K-file or a root canal explorer or pathfinder will find the canal. If the furcation has been entered or the canal cannot be found, the palatal root may be amputated and extracted. The exposed end of the communicating pulp chamber, between the amputated palatal root and the rostral root, is found. It is sealed with a final fIlling material in the same way as the access is sealed, at the end of the procedure.

3. A sharp root canal explorer is inserted through the access hole into the pulp chamber (Fig. 7.3a). If the pulp chamber has not been entered, the direction of the access hole is checked, ensuring that the explorer points to the centre and the apex of the tooth. The depth of the access hole is checked against the outside of the tooth and the radiograph. The hole is then modified to rectify the errors. A little force on the explorer may push it through a thin remnant of dentine, into the pulp chamber.

4. A 25 mm K-file, size 10 or 15, is inserted into the pulp chamber through the access hole (Fig. 7.3b). It is worked in and out against the sides of the access hole to smooth the passage between the access and the pulp chamber. With larger pulp chambers, larger files may be used. Always start with a small size and gradually work up to the larger sizes (size 15 then 20, then 25, then 30, and so on).

5. A barbed broach is inserted into the pulp chamber as far as it will go without force. It is rotated $\frac{1}{4}$ to $\frac{1}{2}$ turn to engage the pulp. It is carefully withdrawn, bringing any intact pulp with it. The procedure is repeated many times until the broach comes out clean. If the pulp is necrotic, the pulp chamber will contain only its fluid remains; there will be nothing with any form to engage the barbed broach.

6. The length of the file required depends on the distance between the access and the apex. For most teeth, 25–30 mm 'human' dental files will reach the apex. The dog canine is used as the example for this procedure and requires the use of 55–60 mm files to reach the apex. The smallest

size of 55–60 mm K or Hedstrom file, size 15, is coated in chelating agent and inserted into the canal (Fig. 7.3c). It is worked back and forth until the apex is reached. This is felt as a dull thud. The rubber marker is moved along the file to touch the access, whilst the tip of the file

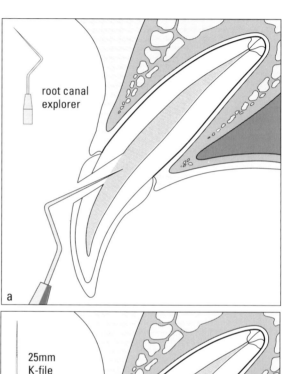

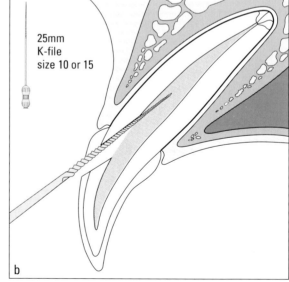

Fig. 7.3 Root canal treatment of a mature upper canine tooth. (a) Checking the patency of the access into the pulp chamber. (b) Removing rough edges from the access.

is in contact with the apex. A radiograph is taken to verify the position of the tip of the file. If it is at the apex, it is withdrawn and the markers on the other files are moved to mark the same working length. In this way, the exact length of the canal is known. The rubber markers may be

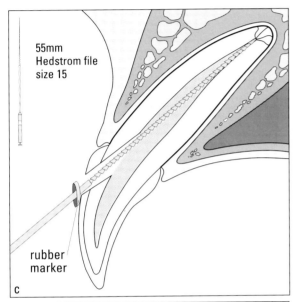

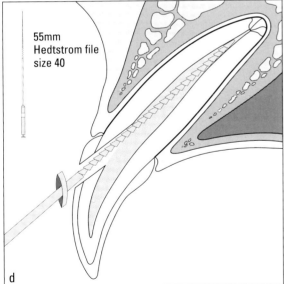

Fig. 7.3 (continued) Root canal treatment of a mature upper canine. (c) Filing the pulp chamber. (d) File cannot reach the apex.

purchased or made by cutting sections of rubber band and threading one on to each file.

7. Clean files of the small sizes (e.g. 20, 25, 30 and 35) are inserted and worked in the canal one after another, ending with the file of the same size as the apex (e.g. size 35). This removes any filings and debris from the apex.

A 55–60 mm K or Hedstrom file, size 20, coated in chelating agent, is inserted into the canal and worked back and forth until the apex is reached. The file handle is held between the index finger and the thumb; a gentle lateral pressure is exerted on the file with the third finger to guide the file on to the walls of the canal, so that all the walls of the canal are filed clean; the fourth finger acts as a fulcrum, resting on an adjacent tooth. Hedstrom files should not be rotated whilst in the canal as their tips fracture easily. Any files with bent tips should be discarded to avoid their fracture in the canal. The smaller sizes are more fragile than the larger ones. The size of file inserted and worked in the canal is gradually increased until a size too large to reach the apex is used (e.g. size 40) (Fig. 7.3d). The file of the next size down (e.g. size 35) is reinserted into the canal and worked to the apex (Fig. 7.3e). The size of this file denotes the diameter of the apex (e.g. 0.35 mm diameter).

Files of increasing size are used to clean the walls of the canal, without reaching the apex. Filing is complete when clean white filings come out of the canal on the file. Clean small files are then used again to clean the apex finally.

8. The canal is flushed with 50% sodium hypochlorite solution then sterile saline several times, to remove any remaining debris (Fig. 7.3f). Recent studies have shown that sodium hypochlorite may be the final flushing solution of choice, although many operators prefer to use sodium hypochlorite then hydrogen peroxide then sterile saline, repeating this sequence several

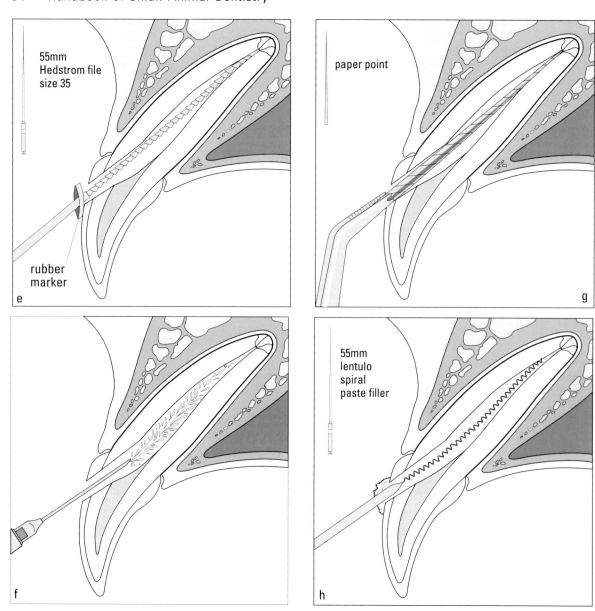

FIG. 7.3 (continued) Root canal treatment of a mature upper canine tooth. (e) Size smaller file reaches the apex. (f) Flushing the canal. (g) Drying the canal. (h) Filling the canal with cement.

times and ending with a final flush of sterile saline. The animal's tissues (i.e. gingivae, mucosae and lips) must be protected from these solutions.

9. The canal is dried. Oil-free pressurized air is directed obliquely over the access. Air should not be directed straight down the canal, as this may force air emboli into the dentinal tubules. Final, thorough drying of the canal is achieved by inserting sterile paper points of an appropriate size and length into the canal, held in locking forceps (Fig. 7.3g). Larger sizes are used to soak up the bulk of the liquid, then a size which will enter the apex is used to dry the apex. Many paper points are used until two

or three successively are brought out dry.
10. The root canal filling cement is mixed on
a mixing pad or slab to a thick creamy con-
sistency (it doesn't quite run off the pad).
Zinc oxide and eugenol (ZnOE) is antibacterial; it takes several hours to set and so
is easier to use initially. Slow-setting calcium
hydroxide cement (e.g. Sealapex) is also
antibacterial and is thought to stimulate the
production of reparative dentine around
the apex, possibly producing a better apical
seal and apexification of open apices; it sets
in 30–40 minutes in a humid environment
(i.e. inside the root canal), but will remain
liquid on the mixing pad for several hours.

The spiral paste filler of an appropriate
size and length is inserted into the low-
speed contra-angle handpiece. It is loaded
with cement, by rotating anticlockwise in
the cement. The loaded spiral is inserted
into the canal and rotated clockwise at
1000–2000 rpm. This spins the cement off
the spiral and on to the canal walls. It is
slowly withdrawn whilst spinning, reloaded
and reinserted. This process is repeated
until cement exudes from the top of the
canal (Fig. 7.3h). The rotating of the spiral
tends to drive the cement apically, forcing
any air bubbles coronally.

Injecting the cement into the canal is not
successful in a canal whose apex is less
than size 60 (i.e. 0.6 mm diameter), as air
bubbles tend to be locked in the apex,
which prevents the apex from being sealed.
Large canals, with apices greater than size
60, can be filled by inserting a needle into
the apex and injecting the cement as the
needle is slowly withdrawn. Hot, liquefied
gutta percha can also be used in this way
to fill large canals. When treating an open
or perforated apex, it is preferable that the
cement is not extruded beyond the apex.
11. A gutta percha (GP) point of the same size
as the apex, the 'master point', (e.g. size
35) is coated in cement and inserted into
the cement-filled canal (Fig. 7.3i). It is
pushed to the end of the canal and engaged in the apex, thoroughly sealing the

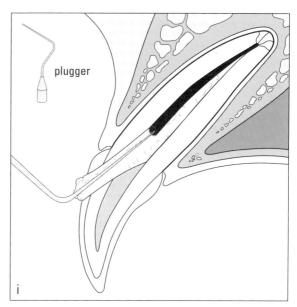
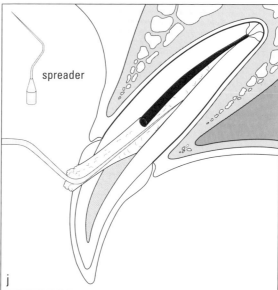

FIG. 7.3 (continued) Root canal treatment of a mature upper canine
tooth. (i) Sealing the apex with gutta percha. (j) Packing the canal with
gutta percha.

apex (rather like a cork sealing the neck of
a wine bottle). Accurately sized GP of a
length suitable for canine root canals (i.e.
55–60 mm long) will soon be available, but
until then, there are three methods of forcing the shorter GP into the apex to effect
a seal: either melt two appropriately sized

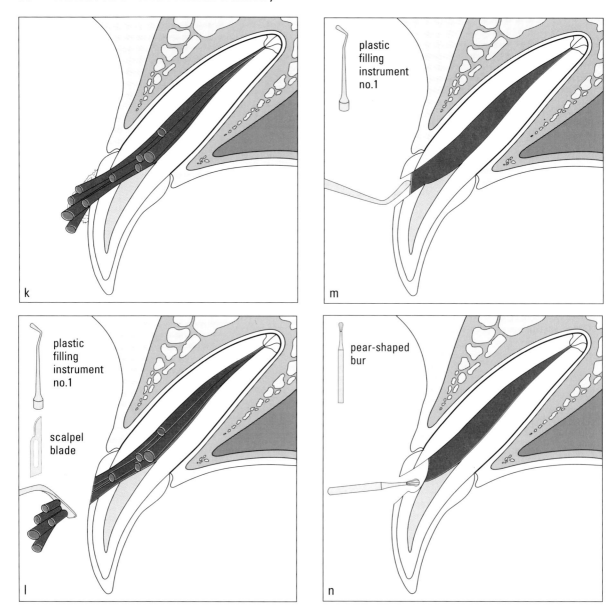

Fig. 7.3 (continued) Root canal treatment of a mature upper canine tooth. (k) Root canal packed with gutta percha and cement. (l) Excess gutta percha is cut off. (m) The gutta percha is further compressed. (n) The undercut is made.

(e.g. size 35) GP points together end to end, preserving the measured diameter end (i.e. the 0.35 mm end); or melt the correctly sized (e.g. size 35) GP onto the end of a veterinary length GP (at present only available in size 'medium'); or push the short but correctly sized (e.g. size 35) GP

into the apex by feel, with a plugger.

12. Further GP loaded with cement is pushed into the canal with the aid of pluggers. A spreader is inserted into the canal and forced in next to the GP (Fig. 7.3j). This pushes the GP firmly against the canal walls, squeezing cement into the dentinal

canals and creating a space for the insertion of another cement-coated GP. This process is repeated until there is no more space for the spreader. GP and cement protrude from the access (Fig. 7.3k).

13. The excess GP is cut level with the access (Fig. 7.3l) with a scalpel blade or the heated beaver-tail end of a plastic filling instrument (PFI) no. 1 (this PFI is made of metal!).

14. The GP is pushed further into the canal with the rounded end of a PFI no. 1, if possible (Fig. 7.3m).

15. A radiograph is taken to ensure that the apex is sealed to within 1 mm of the radiographic apex. If it is not, the whole procedure should be repeated, or an apicectomy performed. Any debris left in the apex will continue to cause pain and irritation, as if the procedure had not been performed. Unsealed dentinal tubules rapidly reintroduce bacteria into the canal, so an incomplete apical seal will allow bacterial proliferation into the periapical tissues.

16. A small undercut is made in the dentine of the access hole and the excess GP and cement burred away using a pear-shaped bur (size 330 or 331) (Fig. 7.3n). If the access hole is already at an angle, a dentine undercut is only necessary on one side, to produce a retentive hole (i.e. the diameter of the outer hole is smallest, so that when the filling material has set, it cannot fall out).

Any unsupported enamel is removed with a straight fissure bur, remembering that in reality animal enamel is much thinner than shown in these diagrams. In practice, the unsupported enamel will probably have been knocked off during the root canal procedure, but it should be checked. The retentive undercut is in the dentine, as usual.

The debris is flushed out and the access hole dried with oil-free pressurized air. If ZnOE was used as the canal filling cement and composite is chosen for the final filling, a 1 mm layer of hard-setting calcium hydroxide cement is placed over the ZnOE

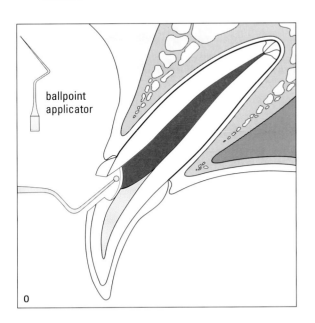

ballpoint applicator

o

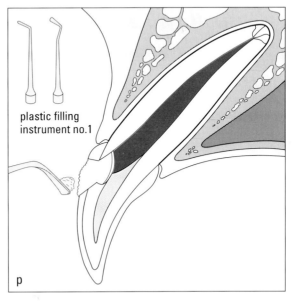

plastic filling instrument no.1

p

Fɪɢ. 7.3 (continued) Root canal treatment of a mature upper canine tooth. (o) Calcium hydroxide cement is applied if necessary. (p) Inserting the final filling material.

to separate the ZnOE and the composite, since ZnOE prevents composite from setting (Fig. 7.3o).

17. The undercut is carefully reburred to remove any excess calcium hydroxide cement, and the debris flushed away.

18. The final filling material is mixed, having prepared the tooth surfaces according to the manufacturer's instructions. It is packed into the prepared site, avoiding air bubbles and ensuring a perfect seal (Fig. 7.3p). Once set, the excess is removed with a long pear-shaped bur (size 331L) and the filling smoothed, finished and polished with a finishing bur (7901), green then white rubber abrasives, then a polishing cup and prophy paste.

Treatment for Immature Teeth With Non-Vital Pulps

Immature teeth with non-vital pulps require special treatment. The dentine wall of the tooth is thin, so the tooth is relatively weak. The apex is open so a normal root canal treatment cannot be performed. Treating the pulp chamber with calcium hydroxide can induce the root to lengthen (apexogenesis), the apex to close (apexification) and the dentine wall to thicken (calcify down), thus strengthening the tooth. An open apex can also be sealed using a surgical root canal technique, where the apex is approached via a skin or gingival incision. This technique does not help the tooth to grow and strengthen. It is not recommended as a treatment for immature teeth. Treatment of the pulp chamber of immature teeth with calcium hydroxide is a modification of root canal therapy and is described below.

Equipment

As for root canal therapy with the addition of:

Calcium hydroxide powder and sterile water

Cavit, a temporary filling material

The following are not required for this procedure:

hydrogen peroxide

gutta percha

root canal filling cement

root canal explorer

endodontic plugger,

spreader

Procedure

The technique is an adaptation of root canal therapy.

1. The necrotic debris, which usually extends slightly beyond the open apex, is carefully removed using files in a similar fashion to a normal root canal treatment. As the apex is open, there will be no 'apical stop'. Radiography is used to identify the length of the chamber and the files are marked with rubber markers so that the chamber is filed to just beyond the apex.

2. Any remaining debris is flushed out of the cleaned pulp chamber with dilute sodium hypochlorite followed by sterile saline, until the fluid is clear when it comes out of the tooth.

3. The pulp chamber is dried with sterile coarse paper points or, if it is very large, sterile cotton swabs, taking care not to leave bits of cotton behind.

4. The chamber is filled completely with calcium hydroxide paste (calcium hydroxide powder mixed with sterile water), pushing it slightly beyond the open apex. This stimulates mineralization initiated by Hertwig's root sheath which results in apexogenesis and apexification.

5. The access or exposure site is sealed with glass-ionomer, composite or cavit, a temporary filling material.

6. The tooth is radiographed and the calcium hydroxide dressing is changed approximately every 4–8 months, as a fresh dressing is more effective in stimulating apexogenesis and apexification. When the root has completed its growth and a closed

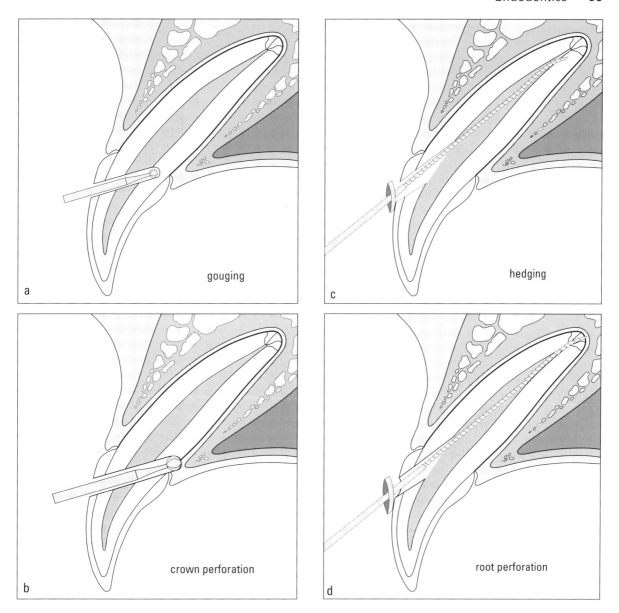

FIG. 7.4 Complications and errors: (a) gouging, (b) crown perforation, (c) hedging, (d) root perforation.

apex is clearly visible radiographically, a conventional root canal treatment is performed.

It should be remembered that immature teeth may well be present in a mature animal if trauma to the developing teeth caused pulp necrosis. Treatment of such teeth is the same as for any immature teeth, regardless of the actual age of the animal.

Complications

During endodontic therapy, complications and errors may occur. These, illustrated in Fig. 7.4, are more easily avoided if their existence

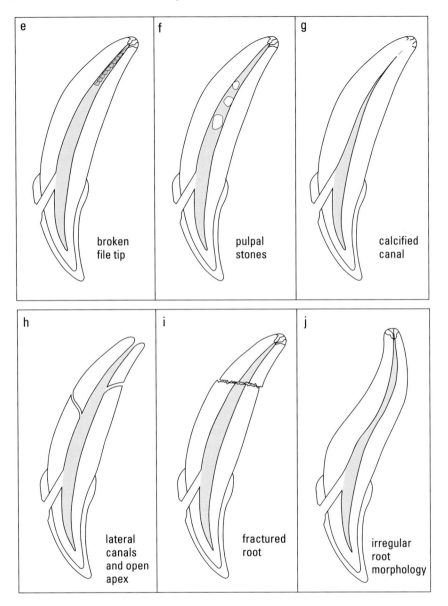

Fig. 7.4.(continued) Complications and errors.

is appreciated, and if the tooth is radiographed frequently during the procedure.

Gouging

Whilst drilling the access into the pulp chamber, the bur may pass through the pulp chamber and engage in the dentine on the other side. This should be avoided by accurately di-

recting the bur towards the apex. As soon as less resistance is felt with the drill, or drilling makes a slightly different sound, stop and check to see if the pulp chamber has been entered, using a root canal explorer. If gouging is suspected, radiograph the tooth with the bur in place. Remodel the hole using the drill or a flexible K-file so that it points directly at the apex, removing as little extra tooth structure as possible.

Perforation of the Crown With a Bur

If drilling is not stopped once gouging has occurred, but continues in the same direction, the bur will pass through the dentine and enamel or cementum of the opposite wall and out of the tooth. With the bur inserted to such a depth at an angle obviously missing the apex, the error is easily diagnosed. The access hole is redirected as for gouging. The perforation must be identified and sealed with a final filling material, in the same way as the access will be at the end of the procedure. Perforation is a common error when making an access into the palatal root of the upper fourth premolar, as described earlier.

Hedging

If the access hole has not been adequately filed to run smoothly into the pulp chamber, the longer files may be misdirected. The operator will feel the sensation of reaching the apex when the file tip is in fact hitting the side of the root canal wall near the apex. If a radiograph were not routinely taken at this point, the operator would continue the procedure as if the apex had been reached and the treatment would fail. Once diagnosed, this error is easily rectified by further filing of the access hole, shaping it to point directly at the apex.

Root Perforation

Overenthusiastic filing, or lack of care when filing a root canal with a barely closed apex, may result in the perforation of the root canal, usually through the apex. Filing is completed to the measured depth of the canal, short of the perforation. After flushing and drying, the canal is filled in one of three ways.

- A plug of hard-setting calcium hydroxide cement may be pressed into the apex on a paper point (to encourage apical closure by apexification), then the canal filled as usual.
- The canal may be filled with slow-setting calcium hydroxide cement (to encourage apexification) and gutta percha, after preparing the canal to the apex; the calcium hydroxide cement is pushed into the perforation when the gutta percha is inserted in the canal.
- The canal is filled as usual, allowing material to exude from the perforation; an apicectomy or retrograde (surgical) root canal treatment (where the apex is approached through the gingiva or skin and bone and sealed from this end with amalgam) is performed as soon as the conventional root canal is finished.

The third method is the most satisfactory. If either of the first two is used, the tooth should be radiographed 6 months later to check for apical pathology or other complications.

Haemorrhage

When treating a relatively fresh pulp which is irreversibly damaged, persistent haemorrhage after filing and cleaning the canal is a common problem. It usually means that some pulpal tissue remains at the apex or that there is severe apical inflammation. Using a clean, long, barbed broach inserted right to the apex, it is usually possible to engage the pulpal remnant on the tip of the broach by rotating it carefully. If there is no pulp left in the canal, 3–5 minutes of constant pressure with a paper point which fits the apex is usually successful. The canal must then be thoroughly cleaned, taking care to avoid stimulating further haemorrhage. The canal should not be flushed with sodium hypochlorite as this will dissolve blood clots. The canal is then filled with slow-setting calcium hydroxide cement in the usual way. A course of antibiotics is advisable. The tooth should be radiographed after 6 months to check for apical pathology. Ideally, the tooth is filled with temporary filling material, the animal sent home for a week on antibiotics, for the inflammation and infection to settle, then the canal cleaned again and filled in the usual way.

Broken File Tip

If a file breaks in the canal during filing, it is rarely possible to remove it, although attempts should be made with a smaller file or a small barbed broach which is inserted beyond the broken file tip. Small movements back and forth may dislodge the tip, when it is carefully withdrawn. The injection of hydrogen peroxide into the canal may also help. However, the tip is usually embedded in the dentine making its retrieval impossible. Using a smaller file, the canal is filed round the broken tip and the procedure is continued as usual, having reached the apex past the broken file.

If it is not possible to file round the broken file, the appropriate action depends on the stage of the treatment at which the file broke. If the canal had been filed clean and the broken file was clean, the procedure is completed as usual, using the file tip to seal the apex by pushing it into the apex. If the canal or the file were dirty when the file broke, an apicectomy is necessary.

File fracture is best avoided. Do not rotate Hedstrom files inside the canal; they are designed to work by repeated insertion and withdrawal without twisting. Do not use files with hooked or twisted ends; throw them away! Insert files carefully to prevent them from becoming wedged.

Pulpal Stones

Pulp stones are calcifications in the pulp, visible radiographically as distinct circular areas or diffuse irregular deposits. An apical seal cannot be achieved using conventional root canal therapy in these situations, so an apicectomy is required.

Calcified Canal

In older animals, the root canal is often very narrow and the apical section totally calcified. It may not be possible to reach the apex with even the narrowest file. The accessible part of the root canal is treated in the usual way, working as close to the apex as possible. This is usually successful, but if there is a recurrence of apical pathology, an apicectomy should be performed.

Lateral Canals and Open Apex

Lateral canals are very difficult to identify radiographically and are usually filled inadvertently during a conventional root canal treatment. If recurrent pathology due to a detectable lateral canal is diagnosed, it can be sealed from the outside (as for a carious lesion) if it can be reached. If it is inaccessible, refilling the root canal with a slow-setting calcium hydroxide cement may induce closure of the lateral canal. The same technique is used to fill a root canal which has an open apex or has been perforated. If this fails or is inappropriate, the tooth should be extracted. An apicectomy is required to treat unresolved apical pathology.

Fractured Root

Fractured roots are of three types, and require different treatments.

Horizontal root fractures in the apical third usually require no treatment, unless the fracture is displaced. The apical segment retains its blood supply, while the coronal segment often receives collateral circulation. A cementodentinal callus develops at the fracture site, preventing pulpal pathology. A horizontal midroot fracture may heal if the tooth is immobilized, but with daily use of the tooth, it is difficult to eliminate completely movement of the tooth which may lead to a non-union with subsequent pulp necrosis. If disease develops, it is usually in the coronal segment. Conventional endodontic therapy is performed, on this segment only. On rare occasions the apical segment is involved; in these cases the apical segment is removed and the coronal segment treated with conventional and surgical endodontic therapy. A horizontal fracture of the coronal part of the root will not heal. The coronal segment of the tooth should be extracted and the root treated endodontically.

Oblique root fracture segments are usually displaced. They can be treated as horizontal root fractures but with limited success. If the fracture line is coronal to the crestal bone, the retained apical segment is treated with conventional endodontics.

Long-axis root fractures cannot be saved and must be extracted.

Fractured roots are dealt with in more detail in the *Handbook of Small Animal Oral Emergencies* by Gorrel, Penman and Emily (1993), Pergamon Press.

Irregular Root Morphology

Using flexible files, it may be possible to treat these canals with conventional root canal therapy. It may help to bend the file slightly then insert it following the curve of the canal. Start with small files and file carefully to avoid file fracture and ledging of the canal. It is often necessary to perform an apicectomy on such canals.

More detail on the complications of endodontic treatment are given in the *Handbook of Advanced Small Animal Dentistry* by Penman, Emily and Gorrel (1994), Pergamon Press, in preparation.

8
Extraction and Oronasal Fistula Closure

Extraction

Teeth are extracted for a number of reasons. These include periodontal disease, caries, feline subgingival resorptive lesions, apical abscessation, traumatic malocclusion, tooth root fracture, tooth crown fracture, retained tooth root tip, retained temporary teeth, supernumerary teeth and client preference. There are many alternatives to extraction for the treatment of most of these conditions, as described in previous chapters, but extraction is sometimes indicated. If the disease process is too advanced for the teeth to be saved, extraction is necessary. Financial and other pressures may lead the client to request extraction.

Teeth with periodontal lesions are easier to extract than those which have normal bony support. The alveolar bone and periodontal ligament are weakened and progressively destroyed by the periodontal disease process, rendering affected teeth more easily extracted.

There are three techniques for extracting the teeth of most carnivores and omnivores. The extraction of herbivores' teeth is descirbed in Chapter 9. The exact technique is determined by the morphology of the tooth to be extracted. In general it is sensible to give antibiotics before the operation and a course of antibiotics post-operatively.

Small, Single-Rooted Teeth

The small, single-rooted teeth are the easiest to extract, although their small size renders them more readily fractured. Patience and the delicate use of fine, sharp instruments is preferable to the use of force, which usually results in the fracture of the root. Fractured root tips are far more difficult to extract than intact teeth; they should not be left in the socket as they act as a source of infection and inhibit healing. These small, single-rooted teeth include the incisors and the single-rooted premolars and molars, whether temporary or permanent, and the temporary canines. The permanent canines do not fall into this category as their roots are large, making extraction more difficult. When extracting temporary teeth, it is important to do as little damage as possible to the soft tissues and to avoid damaging the erupting permanent teeth.

Procedure

1. The epithelial attachment is cut with a new, size 15 scalpel blade directed at 45° to the long axis of the tooth.
2. A sharp, fine dental elevator is inserted between the tooth root and the crestal alveolar bone. It should be narrower than the root, and as fine and sharp as possible, to minimize bone trauma and the risk of root fracture. This is of particular importance when extracting retained temporary teeth or feline teeth, both of which fracture readily.
3. The elevator is gently moved caudally and rostrally around the circumference of the root and pushed apically. The periodontal ligament fibres are gradually cut, torn and fatigued. As the last fibres are cut, the tooth rises out of its socket. Haemorrhage of the periodontal ligament aids this elevation.
4. Dental forceps may be used to lift the loosened tooth from its socket, tearing the last few periodontal ligament fibres. Virtually no force is used, to avoid fracturing the root. If the tooth will not

come out with ease, further elevation is required. The use of force will usually result in the fracture of the root, particularly during the extraction of temporary or feline teeth, where the use of forceps is not recommended. If forceps are to be used, they should have a narrow beak, fit the tooth as closely as possible and be applied as far apically on the tooth as possible. This will minimize the chances of fracturing the tooth.

5. Debris, bony fragments and granulation tissue are removed from the socket. Most will have been flushed out by the haemorrhage.

6. The crestal alveolar bone is filed (alveolotomy) to remove any obvious sharp bony spicules, protrusions or ridges, using a bone file or low-speed bur with saline irrigation. Debris is flushed from the site. Omission of this step interferes with the healing of the gingiva which cannot grow successfully over sharp bony protrusions.

7. Oxytetracycline powder and a piece of gelfoam may be packed into the socket to control excessive haemorrhage and postoperative osteitis. Such antibiotics should be avoided in immature animals where the developing enamel of the permanent dentition may be stained by systemically absorbed oxytetracycline. If haemorrhage is not a problem, the socket is left with its blood clot in place, without gelfoam. The presence of the blood clot is an essential part of socket healing. If there is no bleeding into the socket, the socket is scraped with a curette to initiate bleeding to ensure that a clot is formed. A course of antibiotics is advisable.

8. The gingiva should not have been damaged during this procedure, so sutures are not usually needed. Digital pressure applied to the area with a gauze swab for a few minutes will reduce haemorrhage and compress the alveolar plates expanded during extraction. Sutures are only required to repair torn or cut gingiva. If a flap was raised, the socket and incision are closed with absorbable sutures, as described below.

Temporary Teeth

The roots of temporary teeth are longer and narrower than those of their permanent counterparts. Normally, the roots are gradually resorbed as their permanent replacements begin to erupt. If a temporary tooth is still in place when the permanent tooth erupts through the gingiva, it is classified as a retained temporary tooth and should be removed as soon as possible. The roots of temporary teeth are more likely to fracture than permanent roots because of their length, small diameter and the partial demineralization of the dentine during the initial phase of resorption. With patience and a sharp, fine elevator, these teeth are easily removed as described above, taking great care not to damage the erupting permanent teeth which lie immediately medial or rostral to their temporary counterparts.

It is occasionally necessary to raise a flap to extract these teeth. As one of the aims is to minimize damage to the soft tissues, raising a flap is far from ideal. If a flap is deemed necessary, it is usually associated with the extraction of the temporary upper canines. The technique is exactly as described for the removal of permanent canines, ensuring that the releasing incision does not lie over the temporary canine root.

It is important not to leave the apex as this will continue to deviate the erupting permanent tooth.

Multi-Rooted Teeth

Multi-rooted teeth are divided into single-rooted sections which are then extracted as previously described for small, single-rooted teeth. In complicated situations, the following leverage technique or a flap procedure may be indicated. The removal of bone causes postoperative pain and so should only be performed when absolutely necessary. It is essential to irrigate the site to minimize thermal damage to the bone when using a bur to remodel bone. The upper fourth premolar is the most difficult multi-rooted tooth to extract and so will be used as the example.

Leverage technique

This technique is illustrated in Fig. 8.1, and is reserved for difficult cases.

1. The epithelial attachment is cut with a new, size 15 scalpel blade directed at 45° to the long axis of the tooth (Fig. 8.1a).
2. The furcations of the roots are identified; delicate use of the elevator to reveal these landmarks may be necessary.
3. A cross-cut tapered fissure bur (e.g. number 700) is used at high speed with water irrigation to cut the tooth into three single-rooted sections (Fig. 8.1b and c). These burs can also be used in a low-speed handpiece and are much safer than the cutting diamond discs commonly seen. Diamond discs are too large for use in the mouth and are rather difficult to control; they tend to lacerate the animal's tongue, gingiva, palate, lips and cheeks and the practitioner's fingers. If drilling equipment

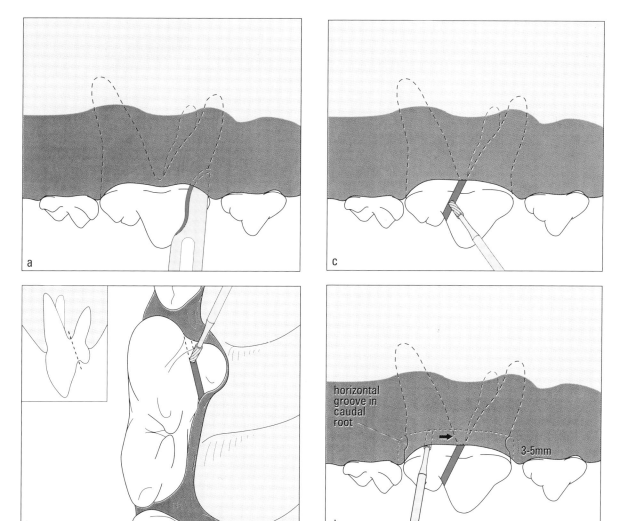

FIG. 8.1 Extraction of the right upper fourth premolar using the leverage technique. (a) Cutting the epithelial attachment. (b) Separating the palatal root. Inset: Section to show location of the furcation, necessitating a diagonal cut in this dimension also. (c) Separating the rostral and caudal sections at the furcation. (d) Cutting the horizontal grooves in the roots.

is not available, a hacksaw blade or an embryotomy wire can be used to section the teeth.

The palatal root is cut first, with a diagonal cut from the medio-caudal aspect latero-rostrally, through the furcation. The rostral and caudal sections are then separated by cutting obliquely from the furcation through the crown.

4. A 3–4 mm strip of the labial (lateral) alveolar bony crest is removed from the labial, rostral and caudal surfaces of the rostral

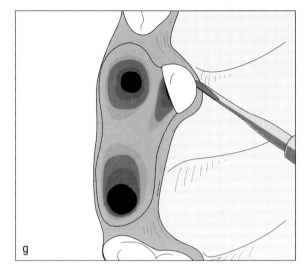

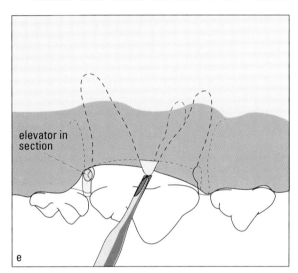

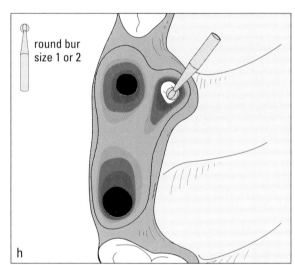

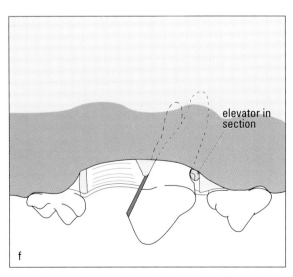

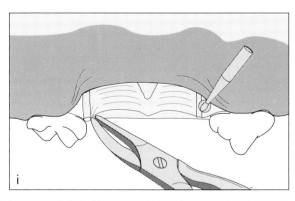

FIG. 8.1 (continued) Extraction of the right upper fourth premolar using the leverage technique. (e) Levering the rostral and caudal sections apart, then using the elevator horizontally to lift the caudal root. (f) Twisting the elevator horizontally in the rostral groove to lift the rostral section. (g) Elevating the palatal root. (h) Atomizing the palatal root. (i) Removing spicules of bone.

and caudal roots using a round (size 2) or pear-shaped (number 330) bur, with irrigation. The gingiva is held out of the way.

5. A cross-cut tapered fissure bur (number 701) is used to cut a 1 mm deep horizontal groove in the rostral aspect of the rostral root and the caudal aspect of the caudal root, at the junction between the alveolar bony crest and the roots (Fig. 8.1d). These grooves act as the purchase points for leverage with the elevator.

6. A strong straight elevator is placed between the rostral and caudal sections of the crown to wedge the two sections apart lightly, to ensure they are separate (Fig. 8.1e).

7. The straight elevator is then inserted horizontally between the caudal groove and the adjacent tooth (upper first molar), engaging the edge of the elevator in the groove.

8. The elevator is rotated to lift the caudal root and push it rostrally, using the molar as a fulcrum. This rotation is relaxed and repeated several times until the root starts to loosen. If the molar is missing, the alveolar bone is used as the fulcrum.

9. In a similar fashion, the elevator is engaged in the rostral groove and rotated, using the adjacent tooth (upper third premolar) or the alveolar bone as a fulcrum, elevating the root caudally (Fig. 8.1f).

10. The rostral and caudal roots are worked on alternately; during the rest, the haemorrhage from the torn periodontal ligament fibres continues to elevate the root.

11. It is rarely necessary to use dental forceps as the roots are so easily elevated with the elevator.

12. The palatal root is then elevated as a small, single-rooted tooth, using a sharp, fine, narrow elevator (Fig. 8.1g). If the tip of this root fractures, it is removed either by further careful elevation or by atomization with a round (size 1 or 2) or long, pear-shaped (number 331L) bur in the high-speed handpiece (Fig. 8.1h). With water irrigation and a good light source, the bur engages the visible remnant of the root and follows it to its apex. It is rarely possible to see the root whilst drilling, but the tactile sensation and the sound whilst drilling through tooth structure are different from those encountered when drilling into bone. Care must be exercised to avoid driving the palatal root into the nasal cavity. As with all new techniques, practice on cadavers is of great help.

13. Alveolotomy (Fig. 8.1i), suturing and antibiotic advice is as in Steps 5, 6, 7 and 8 for small, single-rooted teeth.

Flap technique

In some circumstances it may be necessary to raise a flap to aid the extraction of multi-rooted teeth, particularly if buried root fragments are to be removed. Once the alveolar bone is exposed, the roots are more easily identified, as the bulges of the roots can be seen and palpated. The basic principle of flap surgery is obeyed: the incision line must not lie directly over the bony defect, otherwise healing will be impaired.

1. A new, size 15 scalpel is used to cut the epithelial attachment on the labial side of the upper first molar, the fourth premolar and half the third premolar, carefully retaining the interdental papillae (Fig. 8.2a). The releasing incision is made rostro-dorsally from the middle of the upper third premolar. The infraorbital foramen is dorsal to the upper third premolar, its sensory nerves and blood vessels passing rostrally from it. Care should be taken not to sever these during this procedure. In extremely dolichocephalic breeds, it may be possible to direct the incision just caudal to the foramen, but the final incision must not lie over the roots of the upper fourth premolar. Where such redirection is not possible, the incision is stopped immediately ventral to the foramen, if a smaller flap is sufficient.

2. A sharp periosteal elevator is used to raise a full-thickness mucoperiosteal flap, working the periosteal elevator tightly against the bone over the roots of the upper fourth premolar, caudally and rostrally. The flap

is of split thickness rostral to the infraorbital canal, leaving the periosteum, nerves and blood vessels on the bone, but raising the gingiva and mucosa in the flap. The periosteum is cut immediately caudal to the infraorbital foramen, to allow it to be raised in the flap caudally but left on the bone rostrally. The whole flap is reflected caudally, exposing the alveolar bone.

3. The exact location of the roots is determined; the lateral bulge of the alveolar bone over the roots is visible and palpable. Using a round (size 1 or 2) or pear-shaped (number 330 or 331) bur in a high-speed handpiece, with water irrigation, the labial plate of bone is incised to a mid-root depth (Fig. 8.2b) extending apically 4–5mm (i.e. beyond the furcation).

4. The procedure continues from step 3 to 13 of the leverage technique. When buried root tips need to be found, the area is radiographed and explored from the occlusal surface first. If this proves unsuccessful, a flap is raised and the labial alveolar bone over the root tip is removed, with a round bur at low speed, with copious irrigation. Once revealed, the root tip is removed either by elevation or by atomization.

5. The flap is replaced in its original position. Absorbable sutures are used to close the incision along the rostral and gingival margins, suturing the gingival margin over the extracted tooth sockets to the palatal mucosa. A course of antibiotics and analgesics is prescribed.

This method is reserved for the complicated case as the removal of the labial bone automatically creates a weakness and causes post-operative pain. Where possible, the elevation or leverage techniques are preferred, as the whole labial bony plate is preserved.

Canine Teeth

The root of the canine tooth is large and long. It is normally firmly attached to the surrounding structures. The proximity of the

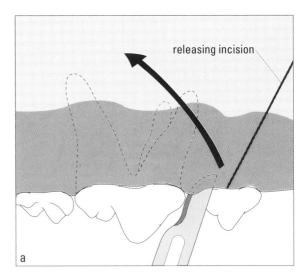

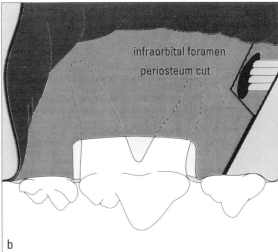

FIG. 8.2 Extraction of the right upper fourth premolar, raising a flap. (a) Raising the flap. (b) Removing 5 mm of labial alveolar bone.

maxillary canine root to the nasal cavity commonly results in the post-operative complication of an oronasal fistula. The mandibular canine root forms a large part of the rostral mandible, which is significantly weakened and often fractured during extraction, commonly with separation of the mandibular symphysis. Unless the periodontal tissues are severely compromised, the permanent canine teeth cannot be successfully elevated as for small, single-rooted teeth, without causing extensive and unnecessary damage to the surrounding tissues.

This method also takes a long time and is physically hard work. The following method, illustrated in Fig. 8.3, is quicker, easier and infinitely less traumatic, with few post-operative complications.

1. A triangular incision is made with a new, size 15 scalpel, severing the epithelial attachment on the labial and rostral aspects of the canine (Fig. 8.3a), extending caudally to the caudal edge of the second premolar, and progressing apically from the rostral gingival margin of the canine to the level of the apex, ensuring that the incision does not lie over the root of the canine, but rostral to it. This is the releasing incision.

2. A full-thickness gingivomucoperiosteal flap is raised, using a periosteal elevator to separate the periosteum from the underlying bone. It is reflected caudally. When working on the mandible, care must be taken not to damage the nerves and blood vessels emanating from the mental foramen. The foramen itself is usually caudal to the flap.

3. The alveolar bone is exposed, revealing the canine eminence (the bony bulge over the canine root) which can be seen and palpated. When extracting temporary canines with this method, a small bulge is sometimes palpable over the temporary canine root. If it is not, the course of the root is pictured immediately caudal to the bulge of the permanent upper canine root.

4. Using a round (size 1 or 2) or pear-shaped (number 330 or 331L) bur in a high-speed handpiece, with water irrigation, the labial plate of bone is incised to a mid-root depth around the border of the root (Fig. 8.3b). Great care must be taken not to damage the root of the erupting permanent tooth when drilling round the temporary canine root.

5. An elevator is inserted halfway along the length of the root in this groove and rotated, lifting the root laterally, using the alveolar bone as a fulcrum (Fig. 8.3c). The rostral and caudal borders are worked

alternately. As the periodontal ligament fibres are weakened and torn, the tooth loosens and is freed. When extracting the maxillary canine, it is essential that the apex of the root is not tipped palatally, as this would perforate the thin plate of bone separating the socket from the nasal cavity, producing an oronasal fistula. For this

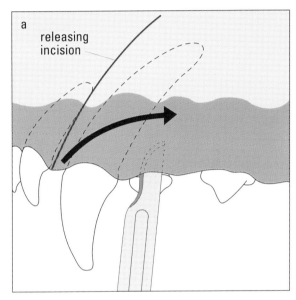

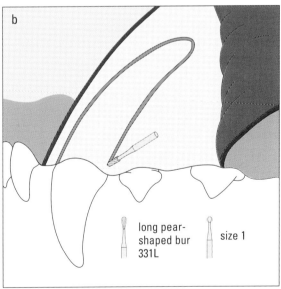

Fig. 8.3 Extraction of the left upper canine. (a) Raising the flap. (b) Burring away the outline of the root.

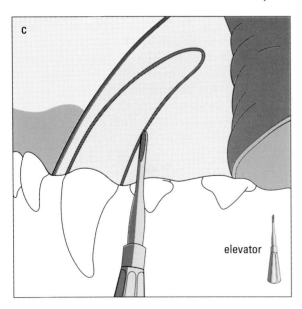

FIG. 8.3 (continued)Extraction of the left upper canine.(c) Lifting the root from its socket by twisting the elevator.

reason, the elevator is not inserted palatally between the tooth and the alveolar bone. Sometimes the plate of nasal bone comes off attached to the palatal aspect of the canine tooth. As long as the nasal membrane is not perforated, an oronasal fistula will be avoided if the socket is closed properly.

6. The irregular alveolar bony edges are smoothed off and all the debris is removed from the socket and the exposed alveolar bone.

7. The socket is packed with oxytetracycline, using gelfoam only if haemorrhage is excessive.

8. The flap is replaced in its original position. Absorbable sutures are used to close the incision along the rostral and gingival borders, suturing the gingival margin over the extracted tooth socket to the palatal mucosa. Digital pressure is applied over the socket to eliminate any dead space. A course of antibiotics is advisable pre- and post-operatively.

Oronasal Fistula Closure

Oronasal fistulae are commonly associated with severe periodontal disease of the maxillary canines and fourth premolars. This is often seen in smaller breeds, e.g. Dachshunds, Yorkshire Terriers and Poodles. On extraction of these teeth, the nasal cavity is visible through the socket, as the periodontal disease has destroyed the thin plate of bone separating the alveolar socket from the nasal cavity.

Oronasal fistula formation may also occur secondary to the careless extraction of teeth, trauma, neoplasia or infection. When the nasal cavity is exposed during exodonture, the fistula should be closed immediately. Sliding gingivo-mucoperiosteal flaps taken from the area immediately apical to the defect and extending into the alveolar mucosa are commonly used, the dead space in the alveolar socker having been eliminated by the removal of the labial alveolar bone. A little oxytetracycline powder may be placed in the remains of the socket, the soft tissue surfaces to be apposed are scarified and the full thickness flap is placed, without tension, and sutured with absorbable material. It is essential that the periosteum is included in the flap to lend strength to the repair of the defect. The failure of this flap and the subsequent development of a secondary fistula may be due to any of the following:

- inadequate or inaccurate approximation of the apposing raw surfaces;
- inadequate scarification of apposing surfaces;
- suture line over the defect;
- flap tension (all flaps must be absolutely tension free);
- necrosis of part of the flap; careless suturing;
- infection;
- or traumatic disruption of the wound.

Once a patent communication exists between the oral and nasal cavities, it is maintained and enlarged by the constant passage of food and fluid. Infection is inevitable. The fistulous tract develops an epithelial lining, ensuring its patency.

The most effective closure of oronasal fistulae is in two layers, without tension or infection, with an adequate blood supply, proper suturing technique and protection during healing. Closure of a secondary fistula is made more difficult by the lack of local tissue, the presence of scar tissue and the persistence of the factors which initially produced the fistula.

Double Flap Closure

This highly successful technique has been modified from the method outlined by Wassmund, a human maxillofacial surgeon. The double flap closure procedure will be described using an upper left canine oronasal fistula as an example (Fig. 8.4a).

Procedure

1. The bacterial status of the fistula is determined before surgery. The presence of bacteria, particularly haemolytic *Staphylococcus*, *Streptoccoccus* or *Bacteroides* species, greatly impairs surgical remission. Bacteriological culture and sensitivity will enable an effective course of antibiotics to be prescribed for several weeks, to render the fistula as bacteria-free as possible prior to surgical closure.

2. Ideally, a full-thickness mucoperiosteal flap is raised from the palate medial to the fistula. The palatine artery is on the underside of the flap and is stretched when the flap is turned over to lie over the defect. The palatine artery runs along a shallow groove in the palate about 5 mm medial to the teeth, as shown in Fig. 8.4. This artery must not be damaged, so, in practice, it is safer to take a partial split thickness flap. The palatine artery and periosteum are left in place labial to a line 2 mm medial to the palatine artery. Medial to this line, the flap is harvested with the periosteum attached, i.e. full thickness. The incision line begins slightly rostal and medial to the defect, progressing to a medial point approximating to the width of the defect (Fig. 8.4b). It is better to harvest too much than too little tissue. The incision turns caudally, parallel to the labial aspect of the fistula. At the level of the caudal extremity of the defect, the incision turns labially and runs to the caudal edge of the defect. It is essen-

tial that the palatal flap is large enough to allow it to cover the defect without any tension. It does not matter how far across the palate the incision extends when harvesting the flap; there is no need to stop at the midline.

3. A sharp periosteal elevator is used to raise the full-thickness mucoperiosteal flap from

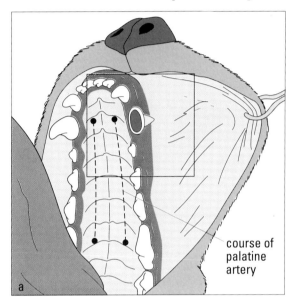

course of palatine artery

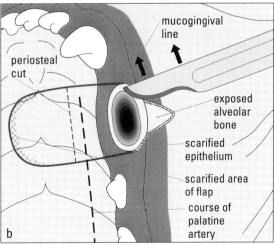

FIG. 8.4 Repair of oronasal fistula with gingival recession beyond the mucogingival junction. (a) Oronasal fistula at the upper left canine site. The box indicates the area drawn in detail. (b) Raising the palatal flap avoiding the palatine artery. The epithelized tissue which will be covered by the flap is scarified, pulling the scalpel blade away from its sharp edge, as shown by the arrow

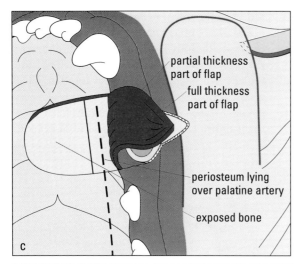

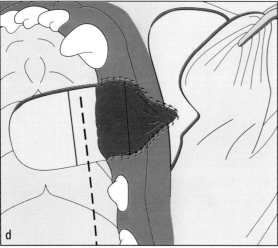

Fig. 8.4 (continued) Repair of oronasal fistula with gingival recession beyond the mucogingival junction. (c) Laying the palatal flap and raising the mucosal finger flap. (d) The palatal flap is sutured in place and the finger flap rotated.

it is scarified to ensure that when the flap is in place, a raw surface is in contact with another raw surface. Without this, the flap will not heal in place. It may also be necessary to scarify small areas of the flap. In the areas to be scarified, the surface of the epithelium is scraped carefully with a scalpel blade.

5. The flap is turned upside down so that the oral epithelium is turned to face the nasal turbinates (Fig. 8.4c). The flap should lie in place without tension. If it does not, further elevation is performed, ensuring that the flap is not punctured.

6. A partial-thickness flap, approximately 1 mm thick, is raised lateral to the defect. The incision begins at the caudal edge of the fistula, 2–3 mm lateral to the defect, at the edge of the scarified strip. It runs parallel to the lateral margin of the fistula, 2–3 mm laterally, along the edge of the scarified strip, to a point rostral to the fistula. This determines the length of the flap, which must reach the most medial exposed area of the palate, without tension; again, too much tissue is better than too little. The incision line is then taken laterally a distance equal to the width of

the underlying palatal bone as far as the line 2 mm medial to the palatine artery. The periosteum is cut along this line taking great care not to damage the flap. The remainder of the flap is raised using the periosteal elevator, but leaving the periosteum and the palatine artery on the palatal bone. Do not push the elevator through into the fistula.

4. If there is any epithelial tissue which would be covered by the flap (e.g. attached gingiva on the lateral margin of the fistula),

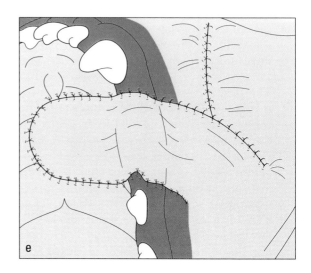

Fig. 8.4 (continued) Repair of oronasal fistula with gingival recession beyond the mucogingival junction. (e) The mucosal finger flap and its donor site are sutured.

the palatal donor site, then caudally, parallel to the lateral margin of the fistula, as far as the level of the caudal extremity of the fistula.

7. The finger flap is raised, 1 mm thick, with a new scalpel blade, taking great care not to puncture it. It is rotated medially over the upside-down palatal flap and its donor site, totally covering both. It is temporarily lain back on its donor site whilst the palatal flap is secured.

8. The primary, palatal flap is sutured in place, upside-down (Fig. 8.4). It completely covers the fistula and is compressed into the site of gingival recession, to eliminate dead space and produce better healing. The tissue will wrinkle to fit into the area of gingival recession. It is essential that this flap is large enough to be secured without tension. Single simple interrupted sutures of absorbable material swaged on to a cutting needle are placed close together, totally closing the fistula. A tightly sutured,

tesion-free, primary flap which completely covers the fistula should be achieved.

9. The secondary, partial-thickness, finger flap is sutured over both the primary flap and the primary flap donor site with absorbable suture material (Fig. 8.4e). It is essential that all epithelial surfaces to be covered have been scarified and their epithelial surfaces removed; tissue will not heal on to intact epithelium.

10. The secondary flap donor site is closed by suturing the lateral and medial edges together, with absorbable suture material.

11. Continuation of the course of antibiotics is advisable. Soft food is recommended for 2 weeks post-operatively.

This technique produces a double flap closure where the oral epithelium of the palatal flap is inside, adjacent to the nasal turbinates, and the lateral mucosal epithelium of the covering, secondary flap remains outside, in the oral cavity. Properly executed, this produces consistently effective fistula closure.

9
Problems Peculiar to Continually Erupting Teeth

Dental Problems in Herbivorous Mammals

A herbivorous diet contains many abrasive substances, particularly silicone, which wear the teeth down during mastication. To compensate for this wear, the teeth of herbivores erupt continually in order to remain in occlusion with those in the opposite arcade. The molars are usually aligned so that their wearing surfaces are furrowed but flat with sharp ridges, to provide efficient grinding, whilst rodent-type incisors are specifically arranged to wear each other down to a fine, sharp, cutting edge.

If continually growing teeth are not accurately aligned with the opposing teeth, they continue to erupt, but are worn down irregularly or not at all. This results in the overgrowth of those parts not in wear. Consequently, food is not properly chewed and so is poorly digested, leading to loss of condition and ill thrift. Food may also become packed in the cheeks and then be lost from the mouth during chewing, a condition known as quidding in horses. If the problem is not treated, it leads to oral discomfort, periodontal disease and eventually starvation, through the animal's inability to eat, or a fatal haemorrhage if a major blood vessel is cut by the sharp points on the maloccluding teeth. Even with a normal occlusion, horses' cheek teeth still develop very sharp edges which need to be filed (rasped, floated) approximately every 6 months, to prevent soft tissue ulceration.

The mandible of most animals is narrower than the maxilla. To improve the efficiency of chewing, the herbivore's mandible moves horizontally as well as vertically, providing a grinding action. The oral opening is small and the distance the mandible can be moved vertically is very restricted. By contrast, the carnivore's mandible is articulated to open very wide, but can move only in the vertical plane, with no horizontal movement at all, whilst the omnivore is provided with a compromise.

The majority of dental problems in herbivores relate to the misalignment of teeth. The mandible is frequently too narrow, affecting the molar occlusion, or too short, preventing the incisors from occluding. Often, the mandible is too small in both directions, producing malocclusions of both the molars and the incisors. Sometimes, individual teeth grow incorrectly.

A metal auroscope is very useful for examining the oral cavity of the small domestic herbivores.

Incisors

Problems

Incisor malocclusion of the domestic small herbivores (e.g. rabbits, rats and guinea-pigs) is one of their commonest problems. The incisors fail to meet but continue to grow. As they are not being worn down, these teeth grow relentlessly into the soft tissues, preventing eating and causing infection and pain.

Treatment

Overgrown incisors need to be reduced in height approximately every 4 to 6 weeks. Alternatively, they may be extracted. Normal food can be eaten after the extraction of all four incisors.

Clipping

It is appalling that cutting these teeth with nail clippers is the most commonly used method, although it does not produce good

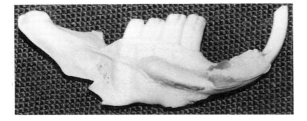

FIG. 9.1 Medial aspect of a chinchilla mandible to show the length of the incisor root.

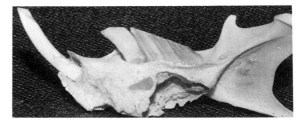

FIG. 9.2 Medial aspect of a chinchilla mandible with osteomyelitis from an incisor root abscess.

long-term results. An incisor will often split when cut in this way, producing a long axis fracture which may reach the apex. Apart from the discomfort this causes, infection can now enter the tooth and track down to the apex, where an apical abscess can form. Incisor roots are very long; the apex of the incisor is found about halfway along the mandible (Fig. 9.1). So, if an abscess develops, it is often mistakenly thought to involve the molars (Fig. 9.2). Cutting teeth with clippers also creates a sharp, jagged edge which may lacerate the tongue and other soft tissues.

Drilling

A more satisfactory method of reducing the height of overgrown incisors is to use a high-speed drill, which cuts cleanly through the teeth, without splitting or splintering, leaving a clean, smooth surface. Preferably with the animal sedated or anaesthetized, the affected teeth are cut with a small tapered fissure bur (no. 699) at high speed, with water coolant, 2–3 mm above the gingiva. The lips and tongue are easily lacerated; ensure they are reliably held out of the way. The bur is angled to produce a bevelled top to the incisors similar to the angle of wear of normal rodent-type incisors. If the incisors are only just out of occlusion, it is sometimes possible to angle their occlusal surfaces so that they do occlude, which may pull them into the correct alignment. If the teeth are completely maloccluded, they are cut as short as possible to prolong the interval between trimmings. As the teeth were not in occlusion before they were cut, cutting them so short that they are vertically out of occlusion

will not exacerbate the situation. However, the pulp is frequently exposed when the teeth are cut. With continually erupting incisors, this rarely causes the abscessation one might expect.

If a high-speed drill is not available, a low-speed drill will cut the teeth, but care must be taken not to allow the bur to 'walk' off the teeth and plenty of cooling water or saline irrigation must be used. Even the careful use of a hacksaw blade or an embryotomy wire is preferable to trimming teeth with nail clippers.

Realignment

As described above, minor incisor malocclusions can sometimes be corrected by bevelled trimming. More severely misaligned incisors may be pushed or pulled into their correct position by digital pressure. At least one hour per day needs to be devoted to applying digital pressure to the affected teeth. If the teeth are grossly misaligned, this is unlikely to be successful. If only one incisor is out of alignment, do not be tempted to ligate the two together, as this usually results in the misalignment of both incisors, rather than the correction of one. The only safe method is firm digital pressure for as much time as possible.

Extraction

Extracting the misaligned incisors of the small domestic herbivores is difficult but can provide a permanent treatment for the problem. If repeated tooth shortening operations prove unsatisfactory, the removal of the affected teeth is a viable alternative. Without incisors, normal food, cut into small pieces can be eaten. Rabbits use their prehensile lips to pick up the food which is then passed to the cheek teeth for mastication.

1. Under a general anaesthetic, radiographs of the head are taken to assess the roots of all the teeth.
2. A small, sharp, straight elevator or root tip pick with a working end 1 mm wide is inserted into the periodontal ligament of one of the incisors. It is worked around the tooth, gradually breaking down the periodontal ligament, paying particular attention to the medial area of the ligament. Firm, gentle pressure is used, but excessive leverage is avoided as these teeth are exceptionally brittle.
3. When the elevator has been worked all round the tooth as deeply as possible, it is inserted between the incisors and pushed as far apically as it will go. It is gently wiggled and rotated. The tooth will be visibly loose when sufficient ligament has been broken down for the tooth to be removed.
4. Fingers or small extraction forceps are used gently to pull the tooth in the direction of growth, out of its socket. The lower incisors are usually extracted first, the loosened tooth being gently pulled upwards and inwards towards the mouth. The loosened upper incisors are pulled inwards with a little downward movement, as these teeth are very curved.
5. Rabbits have small peg teeth behind the upper incisors which are often broken during the removal of the upper incisors. It is wise to extract the peg teeth before the upper incisors. These teeth have small, straight roots and are easy to remove with the small, sharp, straight elevator or root tip pick.
6. If the teeth are removed entirely, the tip of the root is open and soft. If a tooth root is fractured, it may be necessary to wait for the tooth to grow again in 6–8 weeks, then repeat the extraction procedure. If the tooth does not regrow because of tooth root inflammation or infection, it should be removed surgically.

7. If infection is suspected, the sockets are swabbed for culture and sensitivity. The sockets are flushed with 0.2% w/v chlorhexidine gluconate solution. Topical antibiotics may be applied to the opening, but the sockets are not packed.
8. A 10 day course of antibiotics (e.g. trimethoprim) is prescribed post-operatively as a routine. If there is evidence of infection, the antibiotic of choice will depend on the result of the culture and sensitivity test; a 3 week course is recommended.
9. Analgesics may be necessary, but usually the animals are eating within hours of recovery from the anaesthetic.
10. The extraction site should be completely healed in 7–10 days.

Molars

Problems

When the mandible is too narrow (excessive anisognathism), the molars cannot occlude properly (Fig. 9.3). Commonly, the lingual part of the occlusal surface of the maxillary molars is in occlusion with the labial part of the mandibular molars, and is worn down, but the labial part of the occlusal surface of the maxillary molars and the lingual part of the mandibular molars are not in occlusion and are therefore not worn down. Sometimes the anisognathism is so severe that the molars completely fail to occlude. Regardless of the degree of occlusion, the teeth continue to erupt. The unworn areas grow into the soft tissue of the opposing arcade. The lateral excursion of the mandible during mastication frequently results in the partial wear of the occlusal surface of mildly maloccluded molars, producing sharp edges and points. Particularly in the horse, but also in other herbivores, sharp hooks may form on the rostral and caudal extremities of the row of molars, if they are maloccluded in the rostro-caudal direction. All these sharp projections can cut the soft tissues during mastication. This can be fatal if a major blood vessel is cut, but is always painful, causing periodontitis and dysphagia.

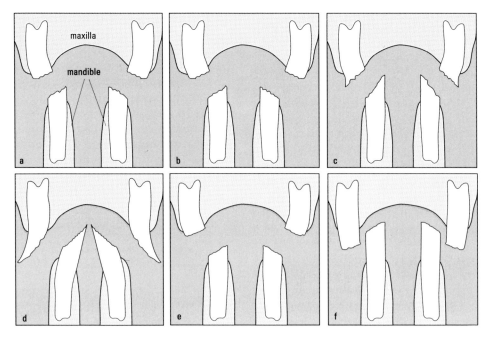

FIG. 9.3 Vertical sections showing molar occlusion, malocclusion and the progression of the anisognathic bite. (a) Normal. (b) Anisognathism: initial stage. (c) Anisognathism: partially worn producing sharp edges. (d) Anisognathism: worn to produce sharp edges, a curved occlusal surface and an abnormal direction of growth. (e) Severe anisognathism: the molars do not occlude at all. (f) Severe anisognathism; the unworn molars continue to erupt.

The abnormal stresses imposed on these misaligned molars may cause them to grow in a curve, the maxillary molars curving out towards the cheeks and the mandibular molars curving inwards (Fig. 9.4). The sharp edges created by the ensuing abnormal wear cut both the tongue and the cheeks, whilst the inward curving of the mandibular molars may trap the tongue. A complication of this situation has been seen in chinchillas, but probably occurs in other species as well. The roots of the maxillary molars invade the orbit and there are corresponding mandibular swellings. It is thought that this may be the result of the abnormal masticatory stresses imposed on these misaligned molars weakening the periodontal structures. This allows the molars to be pushed apically into the maxillary and mandibular bone. The roots of the maxillary molars rapidly encroach on the orbit (Fig. 9.5), whilst the apical movement of the mandibular molars produces exostoses on the ventral border of the mandible (Fig. 9.6). Clinically, the symptoms of

the chinchilla anisognathism are:
- excessive salivation
- drooling
- a wet chin
- wetness around the eyes
- palpable mandibular swellings
- often accompanied by weight loss

The abnormal forces on the periodontal structures result in their weakening, with increased tooth mobility and susceptibility to infection and periodontal disease. Infection proceeds apically, producing apical abscesses and osteomyelitis. This weakens the bone, exacerbating the tendency for the maxillary molars to migrate into the orbit and the mandible to fracture.

Treatment

Filing

The molars are filed to their correct shape, eliminating all the sharp spicules, points and

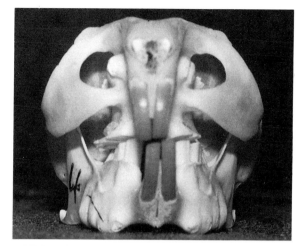

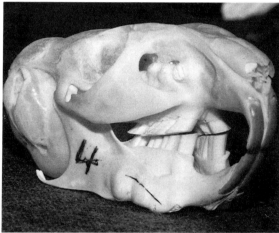

Fig. 9.4 Curved growth of the molars in an anisognathic chinchilla. Protrusion of the maxillary molar roots into the orbit is also visible.

edges protruding beyond the occlusal plane. This is known as occlusal equilibration and has long been recognized as essential for most horses, when it is usually performed without anaesthesia. As small herbivores are not always so cooperative, anaesthesia is often necessary. Frequent and regular filing before the onset of periodontal disease should prevent its progress.

Extraction

If severe periodontal disease has developed, the extraction of the worst affected teeth and those opposing them, in the opposite arcade, seems to delay the course of the disease. It is essential to remove opposing teeth as

unopposed teeth will continue to erupt into the opposite arcade.

As the mouth of a herbivore cannot be opened wide enough to extract the molars from an intraoral approach, these teeth are extracted extraorally through a bucotomy.

Having prepared the skin for surgery, a horizontal incision is made in the cheek, mid-face. It is deepened until the buccal mucosa is incised. The tongue and molars are clearly visible through the bucotomy. The teeth at the focal point of the lesion are identified. They will be the most tipped or loose, possibly with evidence of periodontal disease. If there is any doubt, a radiograph will verify the situation.

A fine, sharp elevator is inserted between the alveolar bone and the tooth root. Gradually

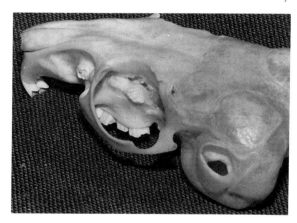

Fig. 9.5 The roots of the maxillary molars entering the orbit of an anisognathic chinchilla.

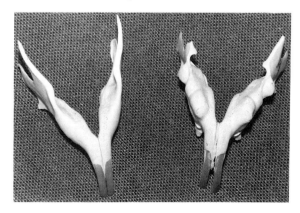

Fig. 9.6 Ventral aspect of two chinchilla mandibles. Left: Normal. Right: Bony swellings housing the roots of the mandibular molars; the rostral roots are visible through small fractures in the swellings.

the remaining periodontal ligament fibres are cut. A small pair of forceps may be used to ease out the loosened tooth. The opposing tooth is then extracted in a similar fashion. The maxillary molars are usually deviated buccally. Once elevated, these teeth are rotated outwards for removal. The mandibular molars are usually tipped lingually so, after elevation, the loosened molars are pushed and lifted lingually, then removed from the buccal cavity. Oxytetracycline powder is packed into the sockets followed by a gelfoam plug to control haemorrhage. It is rarely possible to suture the gingiva in these cases. The buccal mucosa and musculature are sutured with absorbable material, and the skin closed in the usual way. Post-operatively, parenteral oxytetracycline is advisable for one week. Soft food should be fed for at least a week.

Aetiology

The aetiology of the malocclusion is thought to be genetic. In many breeds, there has been excessive line breeding and inbreeding which tends to produce weaknesses. In nature, affected animals would not survive. Without the malocclusions, herbivores rarely suffer from periodontal disease.

Prevention

Since this anisognathism is of genetic origin, the only means of improving the situation is to use only animals with sound occlusion for breeding. Contrary to popular belief, there is nothing that can be fed to affected animals to cure the malocclusion.

Index